# Mental Health - Preventive Strategies

*Edited by Adilson Marques,*
*Margarida Gaspar de Matos*
*and Hugo Sarmento*

Published in London, United Kingdom

Mental Health - Preventive Strategies
http://dx.doi.org/10.5772/intechopen.100962
Edited by Adilson Marques, Margarida Gaspar de Matos and Hugo Sarmento

Contributors
Abdihakim Mahamud Isse, Miyuki Matsumoto, Michiko Ishikawa, Sadananda Reddy, Yakup Zühtü Birinci, Teodora Safiye, Medo Gutić, Ardea Milidrag, Milena Zlatanović, Branimir Radmanović, Chinwe Christopher Obuaku-Igwe, Adolfo J. J. Cangas, Cristina Méndez-Aguado, María Jesús Lirola, Juan Leandro Cerezuela, Andrés López-Pardo, Adilson Marques, Margarida Gaspar de Matos, Cátia Branquinho, Tania Gaspar, Catarina Noronha, Bárbara Moraes, Fábio Botelho Guedes, Ana Cerqueira, Marina Carvalho, Osvaldo Santos, Nuno Neto Rodrigues, Priscila Marconcin, Élvio Rúbio Gouveia, Marcelo de Maio Nascimento, Gerson Ferrari



First published in London, United Kingdom, 2023 by IntechOpen
IntechOpen is the global imprint of INTECHOPEN LIMITED, registered in England and Wales, registration number: 11086078, 5 Princes Gate Court, London, SW7 2QJ, United Kingdom

British Library Cataloguing-in-Publication Data
A catalogue record for this book is available from the British Library

Additional hard and PDF copies can be obtained from orders@intechopen.com

Mental Health - Preventive Strategies
Edited by Adilson Marques, Margarida Gaspar de Matos and Hugo Sarmento
p. cm.
Print ISBN 978-1-80355-924-7
Online ISBN 978-1-80355-925-4
eBook (PDF) ISBN 978-1-80355-926-1

# Meet the editors

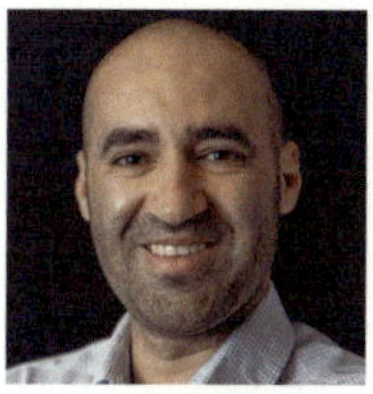

Adilson Marques is a professor at the University of Lisbon, Portugal. He holds bachelor's and master's degrees in Physical Education, a master's degree in Public Health, and a Ph.D. in Sciences of Education, Sports Science, and Health Sciences. Dr. Marques was a physical education teacher for nine years. His main research interest is health promotion. He has recently studied the relationship between physical activity, fitness, and mental health. He has published several international peer-reviewed articles and has been an investigator in several research projects. He is a reviewer for several scientific journals in the field of sports science and health promotion. He is a member of the National Physical Activity Promotion Program at the Portuguese Ministry of Health.

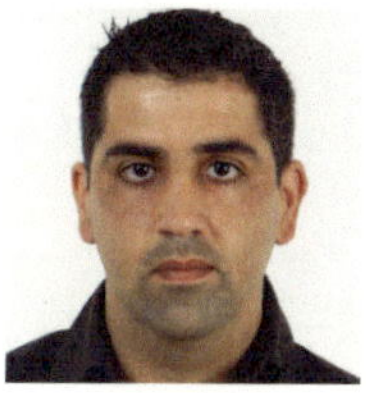

Hugo Sarmento, Ph.D., is an assistant professor at the University of Coimbra, Portugal. He is the head of the master's program in Youth Sports Training. Dr. Sarmento researches sport expertise and talent development following an ecological dynamics approach. He has also conducted studies in performance analysis, training load monitoring, match analysis, small-sided and conditioned games, and physical activity and health. He has published more than 150 international peer-reviewed original articles. Additionally, he is a member of twelve editorial boards of international scientific journals.

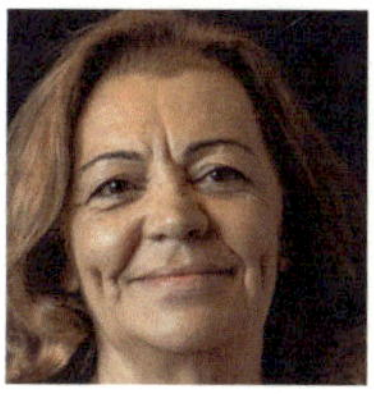

Margarida Gaspar de Matos is a clinical and health psychologist. She is a full professor at the University of Lisbon, Portugal, with a habilitation in International Health. She is the coordinator of G2 – Supportive Environments of the Environmental Health Institute, Faculty of Medicine, University of Lisbon. She is on the Board of Promotion and Prevention of the European Federation of Psychologists' Association (EFPA) representing the Order of Portuguese Psychologists and the Steering Committee of the European Public Health Association/Child and Adolescent Public Health (EUPHA/CAPH). She is a member of the European Monitoring Centre for Drugs and Drug Addiction (EMCDDA) and the coordinator of several national and international projects promoting children's and young people's health. She is part of the coordination team of the international network of Health Behaviour in School-aged Children (HBSC), where she coordinates the Planetary Health Group.

# Contents

# Preface

About 10% of the world's population is estimated to have some type of mental health disorder. Among the most common mental health disorders, anxiety and depression stand out. Until recently, little attention was paid to mental health problems. However, due to its magnitude and associated health costs, it has become clear that this public health problem needs special attention.

People with mental health problems usually resort to pharmacological and psychotherapeutic help. However, these people often do not follow the recommendations of clinicians and therapists, and the associated costs for their treatment are usually high. Thus, the best way to approach the problem is to prevent it through measures that enable people to develop resilience strategies and overcome situations that can result in mental health problems.

This book seeks to contribute to the prevention of mental health problems. It is composed of several multidisciplinary contributions from researchers worldwide. Chapters address topics such as the relationship between smoking and mental health, how management style can have an impact on the mental health of students, the effectiveness of mental health first aid programs for young people, the impact of the COVID-19 pandemic on mental health and resilience development, the relationship between physical activity and mental health, and the role of physical activity in neurotrophic factors.

We hope this book serves to expand knowledge about mental health and leads to the development of strategies to promote mental well-being.

**Adilson Marques and Margarida Gaspar de Matos**
Professor,
University of Lisbon,
Lisbon, Portugal

**Hugo Sarmento**
Assistant Professor,
University of Coimbra,
Coimbra, Portugal

Chapter 1

# Smoking and the Association with Mental Health

*Abdihakim Mahamud Isse*

## Abstract

Tobacco use is the largest single cause of preventable mortality and morbidity worldwide and it is strongly associated with a variety of mental illnesses. Smoking is considered as a modifiable risk factor that has a significant impact on physical health, including lung diseases, cardiovascular disease, peptic ulcer disease, reproductive problems, and diminishment of bone minerals. Additionally, smoking is a major global public health issue and mortality is estimated to be around 6 million people per year. The prevalence of smoking in people with mental illness can range from 50 to 85%, and they are much less likely to quit smoking compared to the general population. Nicotine addiction plays a significant role in the maintenance of smoking in people with mental illnesses. Hence, it is important to encourage smoking cessation to reduce the health risk of smoking. In terms of smoking intervention, international guidelines recommend to treat smoking both pharmacological and with behavioral support in mentally ill patients. Furthermore, prevention strategies are also essential to control the harm of smoking at the public and individual levels. This chapter will highlight the effect of smoking and nicotine dependence among people with mental illness and their therapeutic policies to enhance the understanding of prevention and management of tobacco use as well as nicotine dependence.

**Keywords:** smoking, tobacco use, cigarette, nicotine addiction or dependence, mental health

## 1. Introduction

Smoking is the leading cause of preventable morbidity and mortality worldwide, and there are significant health inequalities in terms of morbidity and mortality among individuals with mental illnesses and those without, and the main factor determining this inequality is that of smoking [1, 2]. Smoking is considered a modifiable risk factor that has a significant impact on physical health, including lung diseases, cardiovascular disease, peptic ulcer disease, reproductive problems, and diminishment of bone minerals [3]. Furthermore, smoking is a major global public health issue and mortality is estimated to be around 6 million people per year [4]. Evidence has indicated that individuals with psychiatric illnesses are vulnerable to smoking; thus, smoking is associated with a wide range of psychiatric disorders, such as depression, bipolar disorder (BD), anxiety disorder, and schizophrenia [3–5]. Recent studies suggest that the prevalence of smoking is significantly


IntechOpen

higher among people with mental health issues in comparison to the general population, and further that they are more likely to be heavy smokers [6]. Campion et al. stressed that tobacco use is not only related to prevalence but also the first onset of mental disorder. The relationship between mental health disorders and smoking is complex and different for individual disorders [3, 5]. As a result, individuals with mental health issues struggled to quit smoking because they experience high levels of distress [3]

The incidence of tobacco use among people with mental health problems was estimated to be about 60%, compared to 25% in the general population [7]. In addition, the rate of smoking is double that among those with mental illnesses compared to those without. For instance, in Australia, a national mental health survey conducted in 2007 found that 32% of mental health patients were smokers, while 16% of smokers did not have a mental illness [5]. Similarly, a large survey of psychiatric disorders in the UK found that 64% of those with mental illnesses were smokers, compared with 29% without [5]. People with mental health issues are associated with high tobacco use, high nicotine dependency, and more severe withdrawal symptoms when they quit or reduce cigarette use [8]. The purpose of this chapter is to demonstrate and summarize the impact of smoking and the association between smoking and mental health issues. In order to improve the response to quitting smoking, it is important to understand the connection between smoking and mental illness. This should help to prevent other related diseases as well as reduce the mortality rate associated with smoking.

## 2. Prevalence of smoking in mental illness

Recent literature has noted the significant numbers of smokers suffering from mental illnesses and the relationship between smoking and mental disorders [9]. Furthermore, many studies have reported that the prevalence of smoking is two to three times higher in patients with mental illness than in non-smokers. Consequently, the prevalence of smoking has disproportionately affected people with mental health issues [10, 11]. This prevalence is rising significantly among people with mental health problems, from 18% for people without mental health problems to 61% for people with issues [11]. Besides this, the prevalence of smoking in people with mental illness can range from 50 to 85%, and they are much less likely to quit smoking compared to the general population [1]. The prevalence increases with the severity of mental health issues [12]. In the United Kingdom, an estimated 30% of smokers have a mental disorder and more than 40% of cigarette smokers have a severe mental illness [13]. Likewise, people with mental health and substance abuse issues also have a high prevalence of smoking of approximately 30–35% [14]. A report from the Royal College highlighted that around 30% of smokers or 10% of all smokers have experienced a mental illness that is currently being treated with psychotic medication in the UK [6]. Furthermore, smokers with mental disorders are more vulnerable in low socioeconomic communities; for instance, around 48% of smokers with mental illnesses are low socioeconomic disadvantages while 33% of those mental health conditions are moderate or high socioeconomic class [11].

Many countries have made remarkable progress in tobacco control and have implemented a variety of policy measures to control smoking habits which have resulted in a reduction in the prevalence of smoking over the last few decades, particularly in the European Countries and the United States [15]. However, the smoking rates in Asian countries did not reveal any sign of improvement [10]. Some of these developed countries have identified that individuals with mental illness have a substantial rate of smoking [16]. Despite the decrease in the prevalence of smoking in the general population in Western Nations, it is insignificant in people with good mental health, hence there has been an increase in the difference in the prevalence of smoking among people with mental illnesses and the general population [15]. A number of studies have revealed that the proportion of smokers without mental illness declined from about 20% to around 15%, while the smoking rate of adults with a mental health condition remains stable at around 29% [11, 15]. In the US, one in five people has a mental illness and half of this population is cigarette smokers which results in 40% of the annual deaths among those with mental illnesses are related to tobacco use [17]. Similarly, a high smoking rate in people with mental health problems has a major toll on death and health status in the US, whereas around 200,000 of the annual 443,000 premature deaths are estimated to occur in these populations [14]. Recent evidence also highlighted that an individual with chronic mental illness dies on average 25 years earlier than members of the general population [14]. This vulnerable population consumes 44% of all cigarettes, which reflects the high prevalence and heavy smoking habits in the United States; likewise, a similar estimate of consumption has been projected for in the UK, Australia, and New Zealand [11, 14].

Unfortunately, recent evidence indicates that smokers are more likely to be diagnosed with mental health conditions, including schizophrenia, bipolar disorder, psychosis, depression, and anxiety disorder than non-smokers and the highest rate of tobacco use are among patients in psychiatric departments where up to 70 and 50% of these patients are heavy smokers [3, 5]. Some studies indicated that tobacco use is significantly more prevalent in people with schizophrenia than the general population and smokers with schizophrenia tend to have a heavy habit, as well as shorter life expectancies [3, 11, 18]. The prevalence of smoking in patients with schizophrenia accounts for around 70 to 80%, whilst different studies have demonstrated that the current prevalence of smoking in individuals with schizophrenia is from 64 to 72% versus 19 to 29% in people who are mentally healthy respectively [19, 20].

Likewise, the prevalence of current smoking among people with bipolar disorder (BD) is estimated to be in the region of 30 to 70% [3]. Although some data can be attributed to small and non-representative groups with regard to smoking prevalence, other studies with larger sample sizes produce different findings; For instance, data taken earlier by the National Comorbidity Survey (NCS) indicated that smoking prevalence in BD was 69%, whereas recent data from the National Health Interview Survey (NHIS) revealed a smoking rate of 46% [3]. Despite the difference in this prevalence depending on countries, clinical studies and populations have consistently indicated that the smoking prevalence is approximately two to three times higher in people with BD than in the general population [3, 19, 21]. However, higher smoking prevalence in people with bipolar disorder contributes to both early onset of smoking and a reduced success rate in smoking cessation.

Furthermore, a recent strong epidemiological study has revealed the relationship between smoking and depression, hence tobacco-smoking individuals with depression have a higher prevalence than the normal population [22]. The estimated smoking prevalence among patients with major depression or those with clinically remarkable depressive symptoms ranges from 40 to 60%, thus the smoking rate is

| Title | Schizophrenia (%) | Bipolar disorder (%) | Major depression (%) |
|---|---|---|---|
| Daily smokers | 74 | 66 | 57 |
| Heavy smokers | 42 | 32 | 34 |
| Smoking cessation | 9 | 8 | 20 |

**Table 1.**
*This table illustrates the prevalence of smoking both daily smoking and heavy smokers as well as the rate of smoking cessation in mental illness patients.*

double among individuals with depression [22]. Similarly, many studies have pointed out the link between smoking and depression and the prevalence of major depression have been noted to be from 22 to 60% among smokers [23]. Other studies with different sample sizes demonstrated that the smoking prevalence in those with severe mental illness were observed to be around 74% for schizophrenics, 66% for BD, and 57% for major depression (**Table 1**) [12, 24, 25].

## 3. Impacts of smoking in mental health conditions

The high prevalence of cigarette smoking and mental health issues are a major public health concern and the association between smoking and mental illness is considered to contribute to reduced life expectancy, which results in premature death in patients with severe mental health conditions [13, 26]. Smoking is associated with an increased risk of mental illness and early onset of mental health conditions and also increases hospitalization among those with schizophrenia, bipolar disorder, depression, and anxiety [15, 27]. Smoking contributes significantly to the increased risk of tobacco-related diseases and excess death among individuals with mental health conditions, thus this has been connected to one of the main reasons for early death in patients with mental health issues [28]. However, the evidence that suggests cigarette smoking is associated with mental illness has potentially important public health implications; to illustrate this, individuals with mental health disorders might have difficulty quitting smoking and may face a high risk of physical problems due to smoking [29]. Therefore, this population might need a strong intervention to support their efforts to stop smoking and to ensure their conditions are not exacerbating due to quitting. Understanding smoking patterns in mental illness is also critical to developing effective treatment for smoking cessation and reducing negative outcomes.

### 3.1 Schizophrenia

Schizophrenia is a serious mental health condition that affects feelings, thoughts, and behavior. This is a chronic and serious mental illness that affects approximately one percent of the general population. Smoking is very common in patients with schizophrenia, which indicates a high rate of smoking compared with the healthy population [30]. Smoking is more likely to be involved in the development of schizophrenia at a younger age, increasing the severity of this condition as well as increasing the number of associated hospitalizations [31]. In addition, schizophrenic patients smoke for a long time, and inhaled tobacco smoke extensively, leading to the concomitant inhalation of a large number of toxic tobacco elements [21]. Consequently, heavy tobacco usage can also contribute to excessive mortality in schizophrenic patients [32]. Notably, as smoking is harmful, heavy smoking might result in a more detrimental impact on health; for instance, schizophrenic patients might experience an increase of positive symptoms and decreased severity of negative symptoms versus non-smokers or light smokers [11, 21, 33]. Similarly, a recent study suggests that tobacco use can reduce the intensity of the extrapyramidal side effects of antipsychotic medication and diminish the cognitive deficits in patients with schizophrenia [21, 32]. Another important association between tobacco use and patients with schizophrenia can be linked to behavioral changes such as poor lifestyle [31].

Although the basic factors driving the high prevalence of smoking in people with schizophrenia remain ambiguous; however, there are different etiologies for high smoking rate and heavy smoking in schizophrenic patients [32]. Firstly, the self–medication hypothesis may provide an explanation, which points out that patients with schizophrenia often smoke to ameliorate the negative symptoms, cognitive impairment, and extrapyramidal side effects of antipsychotic treatment (**Figure 1**) [33]. This hypothesis suggests that neurotransmitter dysfunction such as dopamine, serotonin, glutamine, gamma-aminobutyric acid, and acetylcholine, which is a key pathological factor of schizophrenia, is improved, as smoking stimulates the activities of these neurotransmitters via various mechanisms [32, 33]. Nicotine binds to the central nicotinic cholinergic receptors, triggering the release of neurotransmitters to normalize their dysfunction and improve symptoms that lead to patients continuing smoking. Another mechanism reveals that smoking reduces the amount of the monoamine oxidase (MAO) that normally deactivates dopamine, thus smoking increases dopamine concentration in the brain, which could provide an antidepressant effect [21, 32].

Secondly, the presence of polycyclic aromatic hydrocarbons in tobacco enhances the metabolism of antipsychotic medications leading to reduce the drug concentration in the blood, resulting in some side effects and increasing the requirement for a higher dose [33]. Cigarette smoking has been revealed to lead to an increase in the activity of cytochrome P450 (CYP) enzymes, which are a group of enzymes present in

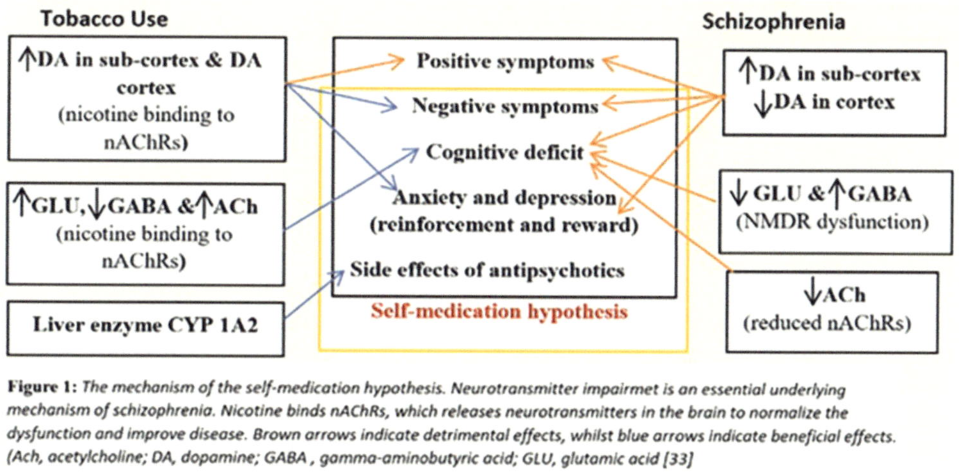


**Figure 1.**
*The mechanism of the self-medication hypothesis. Neurotransmitter impairment is an essential underlying mechanism of schizophrenia. Nicotine binds nAChRs, which release neurotransmitters in the brain to normalize the dysfunction and improve disease. Brown arrows indicate detrimental effects, whilst blue arrows indicate beneficial effects. (Ach, acetylcholine; DA, dopamine; GABA, gamma-aminobutyric acid; GLU, glutamic acid.*

the liver that are involved in drug metabolisms such as clozapine and olanzapine [31]. This is clinically important because it could reduce the efficacy of the drug and lead to poisoning after quitting smoking [21, 31]. In particular, the increase in CYP1A2 plays a significant role in the degradation of these drugs; likewise, smoking also considerably boosts CYP2E1 activity, and both CYP1A2 and CYP2E1 are also responsible for the activation of certain procarcinogenic substances [32].

### 3.2 Bipolar disorder

Bipolar disorder is a chronic, episodic mental disorder that has a distinct characteristic of mania, including mood changes, energy, activity, and concentration [34]. There are two types of bipolar disorder: bipolar I, defined as mania alternating with depression, and bipolar II, described as mild mania or hypomania alternating with major depression [34]. Smoking is also frequently prevalent among people with bipolar disorder, who show a higher prevalence of smoking and a lower rate of smoking cessation than the general population and which leads to poor health-related outcomes; for example, the patients with BD can die up to three decades earlier in comparison to the general population [35]. Despite the high rate of comorbidity and related mortality, a recent study focused on smoking individuals with bipolar disorder and examined the relationship between clinical symptoms and public health consequences: including mood symptoms, quality of life, suicidal behavior, and pharmacological implications as well as biological interaction [36]. Tobacco smoking in people with BD is also associated with higher severity of mania and depression, rapid cycling illness, active illness, higher risk of suicidal behavior, and high rate of substance abuse as well as poor outcomes of pharmacological treatment in patients with BD [34, 36].

Furthermore, it was examined whether these patients could be associated with a poor quality of life, which results in a longer duration of illness and early onset of disease as well as a high rate of hospitalization [36]. The quality of life was lower in BD patients physically, mentally, ecologically, and socially compared with non-smokers. In addition, a number of studies have demonstrated that patients with BD have a higher suicide rate than the general population [37]. Although tobacco use is a strong predictor of suicidal behavior after a major depressive episode in BD, it is not definitely the reason that smokers with BD are potentially more likely to attempt suicide attempts; however, it is possible the aggression and impulsive features may cause particular people with BD to display suicidal behavior [36, 37]. Despite the evidence, tobacco use can be independently related to suicidal behavior in BD patients. There is no full understanding of the relationship between smoking individuals with BD and suicide attempts [36].

The relationship between smoking and BD is complex and multifactorial, potentially resulting from biological interaction, genetic and environmental factors. In addition, the association between smoking and BD can be regarded as bidirectional [35]. Therefore, a possible explanation for the high prevalence of smoking in BD patients is that the clinical symptoms of bipolar disorder increase the risk of early initiation and continuation of smoking. The link between smoking and BD may relate to the reduction of serotonin levels in the brain, which results in impulsive and novelty-seeking behavior; similarly, maintenance and recurrence of addictive behavior have been associated with dopamine and glutamine dysfunction [35, 36]. For example, releases of neurotransmitters in the brain have implicated the pathophysiology of BD and are also considered to play a significant role in nicotine dependence [38]. Moreover, tobacco smoking inhibits monoamine oxidase, which is a potential therapeutic effect of smoking because it enhances the function of neurotransmitters which improves mood and induces feelings of pleasure [35, 36].

In terms of pharmacological impact, smoking harms medication for mental disorders, including schizophrenia, bipolar disorder, and major depression. Consequently, smoking increases the metabolism of many antipsychotic medications through action on cytochrome P450, particularly the CYP1A2 enzyme [35, 36, 38]. This enzyme lowers the concentration of psychotropic medications, including olanzapine, clozapine, haloperidol, and fluvoxamine [35, 39]. Tobacco smoking may reduce the therapeutic benefit of these medications; hence smokers with BD may require an increased dose of these medications to achieve a given level of symptomatic relief [32, 35, 36]. Nevertheless, the side effect of smoking in people who live with BD is considerable, but the negative effect of smoking on such individuals is entirely preventable.

### 3.3 Depression

Depression is a common mental health disorder that presents with a wide variety of symptoms, including feeling sadness, loss of pleasure, feeling guilty, fatigue, poor concentration, and difficulty sleeping or oversleeping [40, 41]. Numerous studies have shown a positive relationship between smoking and depression, where smoking seems to increase the severity of the illness [39]. Despite the robust empirical association between smoking and depression, the actual nature of this link is not widely understood. However, the relationship between depression and tobacco smoking is considered to be bidirectional, in which depression may either cause people to smoke or smoking may lead to an increased risk of developing depression [42, 43]. For instance, some studies have also reported that depression is associated with early-onset smoking, while others have suggested that smoking may contribute to the progression of depressive symptoms [6, 22, 43]. In addition, people suffering from depression may smoke excessively and have a low smoking cessation rate relative to the general population [22, 39]. Despite the incentive for people with depression to quit smoking, they are more likely to return to smoking than the general population [44]. Therefore, it is essential to understand the relationship between smoking and depression and to examine the underlying mechanisms of high smoking rates in patients with depression.

There are a number of hypotheses that have been suggested to describe the high rates of smoking in patients with depression and the reason for continuing to do so, as well as a low rate of successful cessation. The self-medication hypothesis states that people with depression smoke to alleviate their symptoms, thus it is reported that symptoms of this condition may lead to increase smoking [39, 44]. Because nicotine may reduce the symptoms of depression in the short-term, long-term nicotine abstinence can lead to the development of withdrawal symptoms such as a depressed mood [44]; similarly, nicotine addiction may be an important factor for the maintenance of mental balance and elucidate why depression may lead the patient to continue smoking for a long time to mitigate their symptoms [45]. Additionally, tobacco smoking tends to have a pharmacological effect on the brain which is similar to that of antidepressant medications, and also helps the person with depression to relax as a stimulant drug [45]. Importantly, the cognitive dysfunction associated with depression is similar to that noted during nicotine withdrawal; therefore, the depressed smoker is exposed to experiencing much greater cognitive impairment than withdrawal-induced impairment, which considers the overlap of cognitive dysfunction due to depression with the cognitive deficit caused by smoking cessation [46]. This means that patients with depression might well continue to smoke to avoid cognitive impairment.

## 4. Nicotine dependence and challenge of smoking cessation

Tobacco smoke contains more than 4000 distinct chemicals species, and nicotine is one of the thousands of chemicals present in tobacco which is considered to be mainly responsible for tobacco dependence [3, 47]. When smoking tobacco, nicotine rapidly diffuses onto the pulmonary veins and enters arterial circulation, where it moves quickly from the lungs to the brain [47]. In the brain, nicotine interaction with the nicotine acetylcholine receptor (nAChRs) triggers the release of different neurotransmitters, particularly dopamine in the mesolimbic system [48]. This pathway is believed to be crucial to the development of nicotine dependence and other drugs of abuse because stimulation of dopamine induces feelings of pleasure, reward, and positive reinforcement [47, 48]. Such effects begin nicotine-seeking behavior that can cause continuous repetition of nicotine exposure for a long time, resulting in tolerance of some pharmacological effects due to upregulation of the nicotine acetylcholine receptor [3]. Another function of nicotine is to reinforce the release of glutamine from the amygdala, which enhances the release of dopamine, and GABA release, which inhibits dopamine release; hence some nAChRs become desensitized

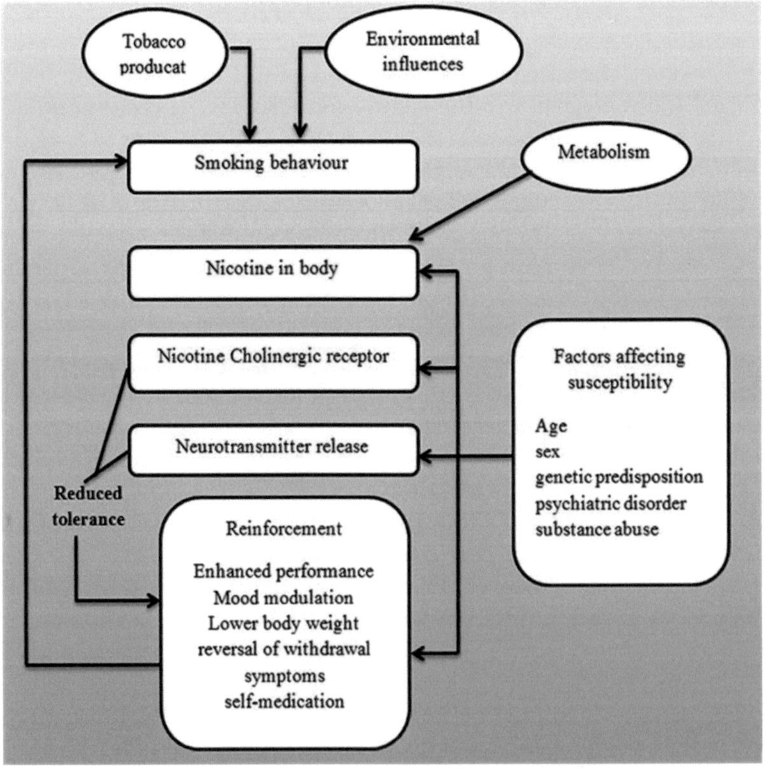


**Figure 2.**
*Nicotine addiction. Nicotine binds nAChRs, activating to release neurotransmitters producing psychoactive effects that are rewarding. Repeated exposure with nicotine results in tolerance in the effect of nicotine, therefore, decreasing its primary reinforcement and inducing physical dependence. Smoking habit is affected by pharmacologic feedback, environmental facators, including smoking cues, friends who smoke, stress, and product advertising. The level of nicotine in the body associated with a particular level of nicotine intake from smoking is regulated by the rate of nicotine metabolism, which occurs in the liver by the enzyme of CYP2A6. Other factors that influence smoking behavior, include age, sex, genetics, mental illness, and substance abuse.*

after long term exposure to nicotine because GABA diminishes their inhibitory effect on dopamine while glutamine activation persists (**Figure 2**) [47, 48]. Thereby, this increases the activation of dopaminergic neurons and enhances the addictive effect associated with nicotine.

Although nicotine is the major psychoactive substance in tobacco use, other chemicals in tobacco constituents, such as the MAO enzyme tend to play a significant role in facilitating and potentiating the rewarding action of nicotine [22]. The MAO enzymes, which inhibit the degradation of dopamine, serotonin, and norepinephrine. Evidence suggests that MAO inhibition plays a significant role in addiction to smoking by enhancing dopamine levels [47, 48]. Moreover, neuroadaptation is a consequence of repeated exposure to nicotine that can lead to the desensitization of nAChRs. The amount of tobacco use also results in almost complete saturation or desensitization of nicotine cholinergic receptors [47]. Therefore, smokers need to maintain a desensitized state to avoid withdrawal symptoms such as anxiety, stress, irritability, loss of motivation, dysphoria, and motivational pain [47, 48]. These negative symptoms and lack of MAO are powerful incentives to relapse; however, nicotine dependence is a combination of different factors, including positive reinforcement and avoidance of negative symptoms [48].

## 5. Methods of treating tobacco use

People with mental illness experience a high prevalence of smoking and they require intervention in their use of tobacco as part of their psychiatric treatment. However, mental health providers have failed to tackle smoking among people with mental health issues because they have previously believed that such patients will not be able to successfully quit smoking. Because there is little evidence on the effectiveness of these interventions to help people with mental illness quit smoking, which is further exacerbated by people with mental health issues being difficult to recruit or retain in clinical trials [6]. Regarding international guidelines of smoking cessation, there are two strategies, supported by strong evidence that comprise pharmacological intervention and behavioral support, that are effective for smokers in the general population [49]. Nevertheless, recent guidelines for a smoker with mental health problems suggest that combination treatment and prolongation of the therapeutic approach may reduce the relapse rate and withdrawal symptoms and it is possible to be effective in people with mental illness [22]. Thereby, cessation intervention with mentally ill patients is considered a combination of pharmacological treatment and behavioral counseling.

### 5.1 Pharmacological treatments

Pharmacological interventions are recommended for all smokers trying to stop smoking unless they are contraindicated such as during pregnancy. A medication approved for smoking cessation can be classified as one of two groups: the first-line treatment is nicotine replacement therapy (NRT), bupropion, and varenicline, which are safe and effective and have been approved by the US Food and Drug Administration for the treatment of tobacco addiction; and the second line medication is nortriptyline and clonidine though there is only weak evidence for the associated efficacy and safety [22, 50]. NRT has different forms, including the nicotine patch, gum, inhaler, nasal spray, lozenge, and others; however, all forms of NRT reduce plasma nicotine concentrations as well as decrease the behavioral reinforcement impact of smoking [11]. Additionally, a single NRT can increase the rate of smoking cessation; for instance, the transdermal patch delivers continuous protection against cravings, whilst the oral forms such as mouth spray, inhalator, and oral strips provide faster relief for cravings [12]. Therefore, the combination of the patch and oral forms of NRT is substantially more effective than the patch alone, and also the combination of slower and longer-acting forms of NRT are more effective than a single form, which are more helpful for smoking cessation, particularly people with mental illnesses. Thereby, the effectiveness of NRT in patients with mental illness is requiring a higher dose and longer duration with more intensive behavioral support [6]. These medications work by alleviating craving and nicotine withdrawal symptoms; hence a patient with a mental disorder should be offered this intervention as with the general population, though with additional close monitoring [12].

Furthermore, bupropion blocks dopamine and minimal norepinephrine reuptake as well as has a degree of nicotine receptor blocking activity [11]. Many clinical trials have demonstrated the effectiveness of bupropion for smoking treatment compared to a placebo; likewise, the Cochrane review also indicated the efficacy of bupropion for individuals who smoke who have schizophrenia, despite the presence of adverse effects such as headache, dry mouth, and insomnia [6, 11, 50]. However, the combination of NRT and bupropion is more effective for the treatment of smoking in patients with schizophrenia, but the abstinence rate was not substantially higher than the rate produced by bupropion alone in patients with depression [6, 22]. Varenicline is a partial nicotine receptor agonist whose 2008 guidelines recommended it as a first-line treatment. It has been reported to enhance the odds of long-term abstinence by about three-fold compared to a placebo [3, 49]. Varenicline works to decrease craving from negative symptoms of nicotine addiction as well as minimize the pleasure of smoking [14]. Although very few studies have evaluated the use of varenicline for smokers with depression, recent evidence has compared the efficacy and safety of varenicline with that of NRT among individuals with mental illness. This indicates that varenicline is more effective for patients with mental illness, resulting in fewer symptoms or worsening a depressed mood in comparison to NRT [22]. However, a further study of varenicline administration in people with mental health problems is required, therefore due to the presence of side effects, it is essential to use it carefully as well as closely monitor use [6, 49].

### 5.2 Counselling approach

This approach is a self-help program involving telephone counseling or intensive Cognitive Behavioral Therapy (CBT), which is designed to enhance motivation and increase willingness to quit smoking, manage negative symptoms as well as prevent relapse in smoking [49]. However, CBT integrates cognitive therapy, behavioral therapy, and motivational therapy. This approach is a behavioral skill that includes support to deal with the embedded smoking habit that may be delivered by a therapist or trained health care specialist [11, 49]. The pharmacological treatment acts primarily to prevent withdrawal symptoms without affecting the positive symptoms and pleasure effect of smoking, and thus behavioral support should aid smokers to deal with the condition [50]. There is also a strong positive relationship between counseling and the extent of abstinence from smoking; similarly, the combination of CBT and medication are important to enhance the outcome of smoking cessation [49, 50].

## 6. Prevention and public health

Various factors influence the uptake of smoking at the population level as well as individual. Therefore, it is important to set preventive strategies to control the harm of smoking on a public level as well as an individual because the motivation of people to quit smoking is different from smokers with mental illnesses. Public health strategies for decreasing smoking among people with mental illness should start to integrate population-based strategies to lower the onset of smoking because most tobacco users initiate smoking at younger ages [51]. Many of these tobacco control strategies at the population level may contribute to smoking prevention at a national level as well as a particular population or individual level [6, 51]. Although serviced-based smoking cessation tends to be ineffective for a high rate of people with mental illness due to lack of contact with the service, the effort to improve smoking cessation in patients with mental illness is significant [8]. However, population-based strategies are successful for smoking control, including, smoking-free policy, media campaigns, age, smoking prevalence among friends, the price of tobacco, and others.

### 6.1 Smoking free policy

Despite the possible barriers to delivering a smoking-free policy in mental health patients, it is considered to have strong evidence for decreasing the early onset of smoking in adolescence, enhancing smoking cessation, lowering the harmful of secondhand smoking as well as reducing smoking-related morbidity and mortality [52]. Thus, psychiatric departments have implemented as they increasingly accepted smoking bans, although these policies appear to have no clear impact on behavioral indicators or compliance; furthermore, it has had little effect on smoking cessation [51]. Nevertheless, the smoke-free policy is required to be implemented as part of public programs that support smoking cessation interventions. Additionally, it is essential to approve smoking-free legislation to attain a high level of compliance, to enhance air quality and reduce secondhand smoke as well as improve health outcomes [6]. This legislation may also alter smoking behavior, increase the attempts of smoking cessation and contribute a long-term effect on smoking prevalence [6].

### 6.2 Media campaign

This is an important component of the comprehensive smoking control program, including a mass media education campaign, expanding healthcare coverage of smoking treatment, increasing the risk of smoking in the general population and particularly people with mental health issues [52]. Many pieces of evidence have shown that media campaigns are an effective way of improving smoking cessation and decreasing smoking prevalence; moreover, media campaigns of anti-smoking have revealed an effective reduction in tobacco use among the general population [6, 51]. Recently, the UK government has invested in an anti-smoking campaign focused on the health risk of smoking and the hazard of passive smoking because tobacco industries and pubic-related activities are a source of misinformation [6, 15]. Therefore, governments are responsible for informing the public about the health risk of smoking and providing the right information about abstinence from smoking; similarly, the governments have a key role in the delivering of smoking prevention in relation to morbidity and mortality and implement a campaign focusing on the younger generation [15, 51].

An effective media campaign also promotes smoking cessation, reduces smoking prevalence, and supports policies of tobacco control programs.

### 6.3 Increase tobacco taxation

Taxation of tobacco products is an effective way for smoking cessation and it also has been demonstrated to have an impact on behavioral smoking in the general population [51]. Tax increase on tobacco has induced the desired effect to deter adolescents from initiating to smoke and to encourage smokers to quit [52]; likewise, the efficacy of tobacco taxation depends on the accessible income of smokers, hence the tax increase might have a substantial effect on smoking people with mental illness [15]. Furthermore, tax increase tends to raise the price of tobacco resulting in reducing short-term tobacco use as well as decreasing smoking-related inequalities. Tobacco taxation is more likely to be effective in influencing the behavior of people with mental health issues [6].

## 7. Conclusion

Patients with mental illnesses are more associated with high rates of smoking than the general population and are the main consumers of tobacco products. People with mental health conditions smoke substantially and thus they are more at risk of smoking-related morbidity and mortality. However, some hypotheses illustrate the relationship between smoking and mental health, and underlying factors driving the high prevalence of smoking in this group, including self-medications, shared genetic vulnerability in smoking. And also smoking may play role in the development of mental illness because smoking has an elevating effect on negative symptoms. Moreover, nicotine addiction appears when smokers depend on the effect of smoking to improve mood and mitigate withdrawal symptoms. Despite the benefit of smoking in mental health patients, smoking tends to harm patients' physical and mental health. Therefore, it is important to examine the underlying mechanism in order to understand the link between smoking and mental illness. It is also crucial to encourage smoking cessation because it can lead to significant improvement in mental health and physical health. Smoking intervention that combines pharmacological and behavioral support is more effective in the general population in comparison to people with mental health conditions. It is also essential to develop a program that promotes a healthy lifestyle as well as improves mental health among people with mental illnesses. Nevertheless, further research is required to examine the effectiveness of smoking treatment in a patient with a mental disorder.

## Conflict of interest

There is no conflict of interest in this chapter book.

## Author details

Abdihakim Mahamud Isse
Independent Scientist, Bolton, United Kingdom

*Address all correspondence to: drintifa2014@gmail.com

## References

[1] Mackowick KM, Lynch MJ, Weinberger AH, George TP. Treatment of tobacco dependence in people with mental health and addictive disorders. Current Psychiatry Reports. 2012;**14**(5):478-485

[2] Brose LS, Brown J, Robson D, McNeill A. Mental health, smoking, harm reduction and quit attempts: A population survey in England. BMC Public Health. 2020;**20**(1):1237

[3] Minichino A, Bersani FS, Calo WK, Spagnoli F, Francesconi M, Vicinanza R, et al. Smoking behaviour and mental health disorders—mutual influences and implications for therapy. International Journal of Environmental Research and Public Health. 2013;**10**(10):4790-4811

[4] Li XH, An FR, Ungvari GS, Ng CH, Chiu HFK, Wu PP, et al. Prevalence of smoking in patients with bipolar disorder, major depressive disorder and schizophrenia and their relationships with quality of life. Scientific Reports. 2017;**7**(1):8430

[5] Campion J, Checinski K, Nurse J, McNeill A. Smoking by people with mental illness and benefits of smoke-free mental health services. Advances in Psychiatric Treatment. 2018;**14**(3):217-228

[6] Royal College of Physicians, Royal College of psychiatrists. Smoking and mental health (RCP, 2013) full Repor CR178. Available from: rcplondon.ac.uk/projects/outputs/smoking-and-mental-health

[7] Leonard S, Adler LE, Benhammou K, Berger R, Breese CR, Drebing C, et al. Smoking and mental illness. Pharmacology, Biochemistry, and Behavior. 2001;**70**(4):561-570

[8] Lawrence D, Mitrou F, Zubrick SR. Smoking and mental illness: Results from population surveys in Australia and the United States. BMC Public Health. 2009;**9**:285

[9] Schmitz N, Kruse J, Kugler J. Disabilities, quality of life, and mental disorders associated with smoking and nicotine dependence. American Journal of Psychiatry. 2003;**160**(9):1670-1676

[10] Asharani PV, Ling Seet VA, Abdin E, Siva Kumar FD, Wang P, Roystonn K, et al. Smoking and mental illness: Prevalence, patterns and correlates of smoking and smoking cessation among psychiatric patients. Inernational Journal of Environmental Research and Public Health. 2020;**17**(15):5571

[11] Prochaska JJ, Das S, Young-Wolff KC. Smoking, mental illness, and public health. Annual Review of Public Health. 2017;**38**:165-185

[12] Mendelsohn CP, Kirby DP, Castle DJ. Smoking and mental illness. An update for psychiatrists. Australasian Psychiatry. 2015;**23**(1):37-43

[13] ASH-Factsheet Mental Health. 2019. Available from: https://ash.org.uk/wp-content/uploads/2019/08/ASH-Factsheet_Mental-Health_v3-2019-27-August-1.pdf

[14] Schroeder SA, Morris CD. Confronting a neglected epidemic: Tobacco cessation for persons with mental illnesses and substance abuse problems. Annual Review of Public Health. 2010;**31**:297-314

[15] World Health Organization (WHO 2020). Brief AP.Tobacco Use and Mental Health Conditions. AP BRIEF. 2020.

Available from: indiaenvironmentportal.org.in

[16] Cruvinel E, Liebman E, Leite I, Hu J, Richter KP. Prevalence of smoking, quit attempts and access to cessation treatment among adults with mental illness in Brazil: A cross-sectional analysis of a National Health Survey. BMJ Open. 2020;**10**(5):e033959

[17] King JL, Reboussin BA, Spangler J, Ross JC, Sutfin EL. Tobacco product use and mental health status among young adults. Addictive Behaviors. 2018;**77**:67-72

[18] Gage SH, Munafò MR. Smoking as a causal risk factor for schizophrenia. The Lancet Psychiatry. 2015;**2**(9):778-779

[19] Gogos A, Skokou M, Ferentinou E, Gourzis P. Nicotine consumption during the prodromal phase of schizophrenia: A review of the literature. Neuropsychiatric Disease and Treatment. 2019;**15**:2943-2958

[20] Ripoll N, Bronnec M, Bourin M. Nicotinic receptors and schizophrenia. Current Medical Research and Opinion. 2004;**20**(7):1057-1074

[21] Ding JB, Hu K. Cigarette smoking and schizophrenia: Etiology, clinical, pharmacological, and treatment implications. Schizophrenia Research and Treatment. 2021;**2021**:7698030

[22] Ischaki E, Gratziou C. Smoking and depression: Is smoking cessation effective? Therapeutic Advances in Respiratory Disease. 2009;**3**(1):31-38

[23] McClave AK, Dube SR, Strine TW, Kroenke K, Caraballo RS, Mokdad AH. Associations between smoking cessation and anxiety and depression among U.S. adults. Addictive Behaviors. 2009;**34**(6-7):491-497

[24] Diaz FJ, James D, Botts S, Maw L, Susce MT, De Leon J. Tobacco smoking behaviors in bipolar disorder: A comparison of the general population, schizophrenia, and major depression. Bipolar Disorders. 2009;**11**(2):154-165

[25] Fornaro M, Carvalho AF, De Prisco M, Mondin AM, Billeci M, Selby P, et al. The prevalence, odds, predictors, and management of tobacco use disorder or nicotine dependence among people with severe mental illness: Systematic review and meta-analysis. Neuroscience and Biobehavioral Reviews. 2022;**132**:289-303

[26] Dickerson F, Schroeder J, Katsafanas E, Khushalani S, Origoni AE, Savage C, et al. Cigarette smoking by patients with serious mental illness, 1999-2016: An increasing disparity. Psychiatric Services. 2018;**69**(2):147-153

[27] Gurillo P, Jauhar S, Murray RM, MacCabe JH. Does tobacco use cause psychosis? Systematic review and meta-analysis. The Lancet Psychiatry. 2015;**2**(8):718-725

[28] Ratschen E, Britton J, Doody GA, Leonardi-Bee J, McNeill A. Tobacco dependence, treatment and smoke-free policies: A survey of mental health professionals' knowledge and attitudes. General Hospital Psychiatry. 2009;**31**(6):576-582

[29] Degenhardt L, Hall W. The relationship between tobacco use, substance-use disorders and mental health: Results from the national survey of mental health and well-being. Nicotine & Tobacco Research. 2001;**3**(3):225-234

[30] Iasevoli F, Balletta R, Gilardi V, Giordano S, de Bartolomeis A. Tobacco smoking in treatment-resistant schizophrenia patients is associated with impaired cognitive functioning, more

severe negative symptoms, and poorer social adjustment. Neuropsychiatric Disease and Treatment. 2013;**9**:1113-1120

[31] Šagud M, Vuksan-Ćusa B, Jakšić N, Mihaljević-Peleš A, Rojnić Kuzman M, Pivac N. Smoking in schizophrenia: An updated review. Psychiatria Danubina. 2018;**30**(Suppl. 4):216-223

[32] Šagud M, Mihaljević-Peleš A, Mück-Šeler D, Pivac N, Vuksan-Ćusa B, Brataljenović T, et al. Smoking and schizophrenia. Psychiatria Danubina. 2009;**21**(3):371-375

[33] Fang Y, Wang W, Zhu C, Lin GN, Cheng Y, Zou J, et al. Use of tobacco in schizophrenia: A double-edged sword. Brain and Behavior: A Cognitive Neuroscience Perspective. 2019;**9**(11):e01433

[34] George TP, Wu BS, Weinberger AH. A review of smoking cessation in bipolar disorder: Implications for future research. Journal of Dual Diagnosis. 2012;**8**(2):126-130

[35] Heffner JL, Strawn JR, DelBello MP, Strakowski SM, Anthenelli RM. The co-occurrence of cigarette smoking and bipolar disorder: Phenomenology and treatment considerations. Bipolar Disorders. 2011;**13**(5-6):439-453

[36] Thomson D, Berk M, Dodd S, Rapado-Castro M, Quirk SE, Ellegaard PK, et al. Tobacco use in bipolar disorder. Clinical Psychopharmacology and Neuroscience. 2015;**13**(1):1-11

[37] Ostacher MJ, LeBeau RT, Perlis RH, Nierenberg AA, Lund HG, Moshier SJ, et al. Cigarette smoking is associated with suicidality in bipolar disorder. Bipolar Disorders. 2009 Nov;**11**(7):766-771

[38] Slyepchenko A, Brunoni AR, McIntyre RS, Quevedo J, Carvalho AF. The adverse effects of smoking on health outcomes in bipolar disorder: A review and synthesis of biological mechanisms. Current Molecular Medicine. 2016;**16**(2):187-205

[39] Fluharty M, Taylor AE, Grabski M, Munafo MR. The association of cigarette smoking with depression and anxiety: A systematic review. Nicotine & Tobacco Research. 2017;**19**(1):3-13

[40] Clancy N, Zwar N, Richmond R. Depression, smoking and smoking cessation: A qualitative study. Family Practice. 2013;**30**(5):587-592

[41] Tan XW, Seow E, Abdin E, Verma S, Sim K, Chong SA, et al. Subjective quality of life among patients with schizophrenia spectrum disorder and patients with major depressive disorder. BMC Psychiatry. 2019;**19**(1):267

[42] Munafo MR, Araya R. Cigarette smoking and depression: A question of causation. The British Journal of Psychiatry. 2010;**196**(6):425-426

[43] Slomp FM, Bara TS, Picharski GL, Cordeiro ML. Association of cigarette smoking with anxiety, depression, and suicidal ideation among Brazilian adolescents. Neuropsychiatric Disease and Treatment. 2019;**15**:2799-2808

[44] Ranjit A, Latvala A, Kinnunen TH, Kaprio J, Korhonen T. Depressive symptoms predict smoking cessation in a 20-year longitudinal study of adult twins. Addictive Behaviors. 2020;**108**:106427

[45] Liew H-P, Gardner S. The interrelationship between smoking and depression in Indonesia. Health Policy and Technology. 2016;**5**(1):26-31

[46] Mathew AR, Hogarth L, Leventhal AM, Cook JW, Hitsman B. Cigarette smoking and depression

comorbidity: Systematic review and proposed theoretical model. Addiction. 2017;**112**(3):401-412

[47] Rosenthal DG, Weitzman M, Benowitz NL. Nicotine addiction: Mechanisms and consequences. International Journal of Mental Health. 2014;**40**(1):22-38

[48] Benowitz NL. Nicotine addiction. The New England Journal of Medicine. 2010;**362**(24):2295-2303

[49] Hitsman B, Moss TG, Montoya ID, George TP. Treatment of tobacco dependence in mental health and addictive disorders. The Canadian Journal of Psychiatry. 2009 Jun;**54**(6):368-378

[50] Cosci F, Pistelli F, Lazzarini N, Carrozzi L. Nicotine dependence and psychological distress: Outcomes and clinical implications in smoking cessation. Psychology Research and Behavior Management. 2011;**4**:119-128

[51] Compton MT, Daumit GL, Druss BG. Cigarette smoking and overweight/ obesity among individuals with serious mental illnesses: A preventive perspective. Harvard Review of Psychiatry. 2006;**14**(4):212-222

[52] Prochaska JJ, Benowitz NL. Current advances in research in treatment and recovery: Nicotine addiction. Science Advances. 2019;**5**(10):eaay9763

Chapter 2

# Perspective Chapter: Mental Health Issues of Japanese Elementary School Teachers – The Effects of the Japanese Classroom Management Style

*Miyuki Matsumoto, Michiko Ishikawa and Sadananda Reddy*

**Abstract**

Teachers in Japan face work-related mental health issues, such as depression and adjustment disorders. The number of elementary school teachers taking leave of absence due to mental illness has been increasing every year and is high according to international standards. One of the reasons for this was the workload on a single teacher, resulting in long working hours. The authors believe that the reason for long working hours may be the Japanese classroom management style. This chapter compares the Japanese classroom management style of elementary school teachers with the classroom management styles of other countries, such as India, and discusses the reasons for the long working hours under the Japanese classroom management style.

**Keywords:** Japanese elementary school teachers, Japanese classroom management style, mental health issues, long working hours, over-occupation

## 1. Introduction

Japanese teachers are extremely busy, dealing with problems of truancy, bullying, and the COVID-19 pandemic. The circumstances teachers have to adapt to and situations they need to address have left them feeling alone and mentally overwhelmed.

In this chapter, we will discuss the reasons for their mental state, citing Japanese-style classroom management as one of the risks for Japanese teachers to become mentally overwhelmed and develop mental health issues, such as depression and adjustment disorder.

Comparing classroom management in Japan with that in other countries is useful in understanding how the Japanese situation differs, and what issues it faces. This chapter will focus on India as a country for comparison, given that there are many similarities between the Japanese and Indian primary education systems, despite their cultural differences. These similarities can be attributed to the historical background of both countries, where Western education systems were introduced after the defeat in war or colonialism and applied over existing local education systems [1, 2]. Such a comparison will be beneficial for both countries. For Japan, the comparison with classroom management in a different culture can help clarify local issues. Meanwhile, India's pressing need for elementary education reform can be aided by examining Japan's elementary education classroom management.

Classroom management consists of all the actions taken by teachers to create an environment supporting and promoting both academic and social-emotional learning [3, 4]. While there are numerous definitions of classroom management, they usually include actions taken by teachers to establish order, attract students, and elicit cooperation [5]. For instance, classroom management is also often understood as classroom discipline, which emphasizes on issues like the treatment of cheating [6], and as the process by which teachers create a classroom setting and maintain appropriate student behavior [7]. Proper classroom management improves student performance and achievement [8]. Japan's Ministry of Education, Culture, Sports, Science and Technology (MEXT) states that "Classroom management is generally considered to be managed and developed in accordance with the goals and policies of classroom management developed by the homeroom teacher based on the educational goals of the school and the actual situation of the classroom, and by creating the necessary conditions."

The Organization for Economic Cooperation and Development (OECD) is an international organization with 38 developed countries, mainly European countries but also including Japan and the U.S.

## 2. What is the reason Japanese teachers are over-occupied?

According to the MEXT, 5180 public elementary and secondary school teachers took a leave of absence due to mental illness in 2020 in Japan; in 2019, the number was 5478, a record high.

Previously published data show that the number of teachers who took leave due to mental illness was about 1600–1900 every year from 1997 to 1999, and about 2300–2700 every year from 2000 to 2002.

The number increased in the 2000s and has remained at approximately 5000 per year since 2007 (**Table 1**) [9].

From 2004 to 2016, 1323 school faculty members (615 men and 708 women, mean age 47.2 years) visited the Kyushu Central Hospital Mental Health Center. Of these, 138 (59 males, 79 females, average age 46.1 years) took a leave of absence. **Table 2** shows what the attending physicians judged to be the "main causes" of faculty members' leaves of absence [10].

The results indicate that dealing with students and parents is a common cause of leave for elementary school teachers. In other words, many teachers suffer from mental health problems due to strained relationships with certain students or parents or because their classes are no longer feasible because of these problems, leading to a leave of absence.

How many teachers take sick leave up to a month, if not a leave of absence? In Japan, a leave of absence for public school teachers is an administrative action during which their salaries may be cut. Before this leave, they could take sick leave. In most cases, sick leave lasts up to 90 days.

**Table 3** shows that the number of teachers who obtained long-term treatment of 1 month or more due to mental illness was 8071 in 2016, 8470 in 2017, 9062 in 2018, 9642 in 2019, and 9452 in 2020. The rate of increase from 2016 to 2020 shows that the number of teachers on long-term treatment due to mental illness is 1.28 times higher,

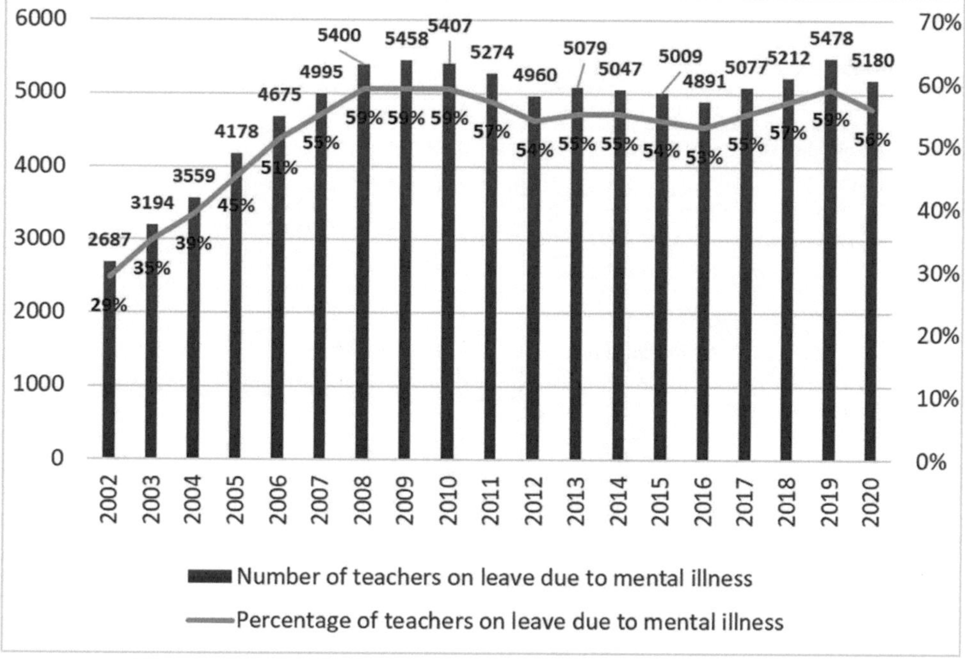


**Table 1.**
*Personnel administration status survey of Japanese public school teachers in 2020.*

| | Elementary schools | Secondary schools | High schools | Special support | Total |
|---|---|---|---|---|---|
| Dealing with difficult students | 32 | 12 | 1 | 0 | 45 |
| Dealing with parents | 15 | 4 | 0 | 2 | 21 |
| Relationships with teachers in management | 8 | 3 | 1 | 1 | 13 |
| Unfamiliar work environment due to transfer | 3 | 2 | 2 | 1 | 9 |
| Relationships with co-workers | 2 | 2 | 1 | 3 | 8 |
| Large overall workload | 3 | 1 | 0 | 0 | 4 |
| Stress at home | 3 | 0 | 0 | 0 | 3 |
| Content of subject matter instruction | 0 | 0 | 1 | 0 | 1 |
| Research classes | 1 | 0 | 0 | 0 | 1 |
| Others (health, nursing care, etc.) | 16 | 14 | 3 | 0 | 33 |
| Total | 83 | 38 | 9 | 8 | 138 |

**Table 2.**
*The main reason for the faculty member's leave of absence.*

especially in elementary schools. The rate of increase from 2016 to 2020 shows that the number of those in long-term treatment for mental illness is 1.28 times higher in elementary schools and 1.66 times higher among teachers in their 20s. This is followed by teachers in their 30s, who are 1.43 times more likely to be under long-term

| | | 2016 | 2017 | 2018 | 2019 | 2020 | Increase from 2016 to 2020 |
|---|---|---|---|---|---|---|---|
| **Elementary schools** | Mental illness | 3668 | 3889 | 4290 | 4729 | 4691 | **1.28** |
| | Nonmental illness | 4134 | 4010 | 3922 | 3863 | 3794 | 0.92 |
| **Secondary schools** | Mental illness | 2155 | 2268 | 2348 | 2387 | 2292 | 1.06 |
| | Nonmental illness | 2003 | 2048 | 2092 | 1949 | 1789 | 0.89 |
| **High schools** | Mental illness | 1193 | 1243 | 1309 | 1329 | 1273 | 1.07 |
| | Nonmental illness | 1378 | 1453 | 1426 | 1386 | 1317 | 0.96 |
| **Special support schools** | Mental illness | 1044 | 1054 | 1092 | 1157 | 1143 | 1.09 |
| | Nonmental illness | 1198 | 1201 | 1153 | 1153 | 1147 | 0.96 |
| | | 2016 | 2017 | 2018 | 2019 | 2020 | Increase from 2016 to 2020 |
| **20s** | Mental illness | 1286 | 1576 | 1765 | 1950 | 2140 | **1.66** |
| | Nonmental illness | 776 | 852 | 806 | 833 | 884 | **1.14** |
| **30s** | Mental illness | 1788 | 2012 | 2302 | 2614 | 2563 | **1.43** |
| | Nonmental illness | 2126 | 2019 | 2126 | 2038 | 2062 | 0.97 |
| **40s** | Mental illness | 2024 | 2057 | 2141 | 2228 | 2138 | 1.06 |
| | Nonmental illness | 1909 | 1893 | 1757 | 1668 | 1574 | 0.82 |
| **50s and above** | Mental illness | 2973 | 2825 | 2854 | 2850 | 2611 | 0.88 |
| | Nonmental illness | 3917 | 3962 | 3933 | 3849 | 3574 | 0.91 |

**Table 3.**
*Number of public school teachers receiving medical treatment for more than 1 month (including those on leave).*

treatment for mental illness. These results indicate that mental health problems are more serious among young teachers in their 20s and 30s in elementary schools [11].

One of the reasons for the increase in the number of elementary school teachers with mental health problems is that although there tends to be a large number of young teachers in their twenties and thirties in elementary schools, the number of teachers in their mid-forties to fifties who can guide these teachers is small, and they are not able to practically guide the teachers [12]. In this case, teachers have no one to consult when they have to deal with complaints from parents or when they are unable to cope with classroom management, which leads them to face problems alone.

There is a serious shortage of teachers and instructors in Japan. The number of teachers who are on long-term medical treatment or leave of absence is increasing, but the number of teachers who cannot replace them is increasing all over Japan, especially in urban areas. To compensate for the shortage of manpower in the field of education, mid-career and veteran teachers have been assigned to cover the remaining teachers, and they have become so busy that it has become difficult for them to provide guidance to the remaining young teachers, listen to their concerns and support them, and take organizational action before the problem becomes too big.

Furthermore, the fact that COVID-19 measures require manpower and additional attention increases the burden on the educational field.

International comparisons confirm that Japanese teachers' busyness is among the worst in the world.

According to TALIS2018, in which 48 regions and countries, including OECD countries, participated, teachers' work hours per week were 54.4 hours for elementary school teachers and 56.0 hours for secondary school teachers, the longest among the participating regions and countries. The average working hours for the participating regions and countries (secondary school teachers) was 38.3 hours. This is not because of the long hours of teaching, but because of the long hours of extracurricular activities, especially for junior high school teachers (7.5 hours, the longest among the participating regions and countries, with an average of 1.9 hours).

The time spent on administrative activities was also long for both elementary and junior high school teachers (5.2 hours for elementary school teachers and 5.6 hours for junior high school teachers, both the longest in the participating regions and countries). The average time was 2.7 hours. On the other hand, Japanese elementary and junior high school teachers spent the least amount of time on professional development among the participating regions and countries (0.7 hours for elementary teachers and 0.6 hours for junior high school teachers, an average of 2.0 hours). Based on the results of this survey, many Japanese elementary and junior high school principals pointed out a lack of support staff and teachers capable of teaching students with special needs and provide quality instructions. However, few cited the lack of teaching materials and textbooks [13].

## 3. Classroom management of Japanese elementary school teachers

The Japanese style of classroom management can be seen as "teaching according to students' difficulties and creating a group based on an understanding of each student's situation" [14].

In a study in which 17 Japanese elementary school teachers were interviewed about how they think about classroom management, the interviews were analyzed using a modified version of grounded theory, and six categories were identified. These six categories are listed in **Table 4** [15].

### 3.1 Data collection and study participants

Teachers were selected based on the criteria that they (1) had at least 2 years of experience as school teachers and (2) worked in schools in the three prefectures to which the authors had access. All 17 teachers had experience in public elementary schools, had come to teach at the graduate school of teaching, and were recommended by administrators or school boards, such as supervisors at practicum schools or in-service teacher students. Private elementary school teachers were excluded since private schools have their own methods and goals, and it is not possible to generalize about them. Each teacher was informed in advance, in writing, of the purpose of the study, that they were free to discontinue the study, that the data would only be used for research purposes, and that they would not be personally identified, and their consent was obtained.

### 3.2 Data collection period

Data collection was conducted from September to December 2017. Thus, the collected data were unaffected by the COVID-19 pandemic.

| | Category | Definition |
|---|---|---|
| I | Understanding children and connecting with children | For teachers to deepen their understanding of each child through their own experiences and also to devise ways to connect with children. |
| II | Understanding the developmental stages of children and dealing with individuals and groups | Understand the developmental stages of children in the lower, middle, and upper grades and coordinate with the individual and the group to nurture them as a class group. |
| III | The will and skills of the homeroom teacher to give direction to the class while also providing special needs education. | The homeroom teacher has a policy for the child's upbringing and not only deals with children who have difficulties but also gives direction to the classroom. |
| IV | Responding to parents on the basis of responding to children | Classroom management, including the creation of the classroom environment, lesson planning, and the opening of the classroom, is a major task for teachers, but it is also necessary to collaborate with parents through the relationship with children in classroom management. |
| V | To develop into a chief through work | Teachers report and discuss their daily work with senior teachers and administrators and are promoted to senior teachers through this experience. |
| VI | A teacher's attitude to learn from failure | Teachers learn from their mistakes and overcome them, so that the growth of the children becomes their own joy and sense of mission. |

**Table 4.**
*Categories of classroom management for Japanese elementary school teachers.*

In addition, a survey of 261 Japanese elementary school teachers was conducted to create the "Japanese Classroom Management for Elementary School Teachers' scale, and its reliability and validity were confirmed [14]. The results of an exploratory factor analysis showed that there were a total of 17 items: 9 items on how to create a group (creating a classroom that gives direction to the individual and the group), 3 items on understanding children (understanding individual children), and 5 items on teacher attitude (attitude as a teacher).

In Japanese classroom management, the focus is on integrating individuals into a group. Elementary school teachers must focus on dealing with each child and organizing them into groups.

In this context, teachers are required to work with students to grasp their situations accurately. In Japan, elementary school teachers are expected to spend time with students not only during class time but also during recess, lunch time, cleaning time, special activity time, club activities, and all other times in their school life.

As mentioned earlier, most elementary school teachers in Japan today are in their 20s and 30s, with little experience, while there are few experienced teachers in their late 40s and 50s.

Therefore, it is difficult for inexperienced teachers to implement ideal classroom management, and various difficulties are expected to arise.

When Japanese elementary school teachers face difficulties, they cannot simply ignore them. This is because the people around them, and most importantly the teachers themselves, cannot forgive them. Elementary school teachers who face difficulties in classroom management try to tackle them on their own because they have little experience and no other teachers to consult. This leads to longer working hours.

In addition, trying to tackle the work on their own can lead to a decline in self-esteem if they feel they cannot do it.

## 4. Classroom management of Indian elementary school teachers

Ishikawa, who investigated the classroom management of Indian elementary school teachers, said, "India is a secular country with diverse ethnicities and cultures, premised on the segregation of people, so Indian teachers are unlikely to have the concept of rising groups" [16].

India comprises 28 states and 8 union territories. Education in India is under the joint direct control of federal and state governments. However, substantive authority to control education in each state rests in the hands of state governments. The union territories are directly governed by the Union Government of India, but it should be noted that they do not necessarily have a unified educational system [17].

In India, the primary and secondary levels of education are 12 years long, that is, the 10 + 2 system of education has been standardized, with 10 years for early primary education and 2 years for early secondary education. However, the structure of the first 10 years of education differs from state to state and from Federal District to Federal District (2009–2010, 5–2-3 system: 18 states and 4 federal jurisdictions; 4–3-3 system: 8 states and 3 federal jurisdictions; 5–2-3 system: 1 state; 4–4-2 system: 1 state).

The National Council of Educational Research and Training (NCERT) formulates the framework of the national curriculum, and each state's councils of educational research and training organize its state curriculum based on this framework.

While elementary schools in Japan are mostly public schools, those in India are classified according to the entities that establish and operate them. The two main types of schools are government and private. Government schools include Central schools established and operated by the federal government, state schools established and operated by the state education departments, and schools established and operated by local governments. Private schools are classified according to whether they are accredited, subsidized by the government, and legal.

Starting with the Compulsory Education Act of the British colonial era, India, has pursued a policy of universalization of education up to the present day. The government's policy of universalizing primary education has contributed to increasing school enrollment by building more schools and classrooms and increasing the number of teachers. However, the policy's emphasis on quantitative expansion has caused various qualitative problems. Many of the children of the first generation of learners, who grew up in illiterate families and had never been educated before, were concentrated in public schools. However, public schools could not keep up with the growing number of students, and, as a temporary measure, unqualified contract teachers were sometimes hired at low wages. In the less developed states, where there was still a shortage of teachers, double-enrollment classes were implemented, where one teacher taught several grades simultaneously, and one-teacher schools were established, where one teacher ran the entire school operation.

In response to this situation in public schools, wealthy and middle-class people, mainly in urban India, enroll their children in unsubsidized private schools that provide paid education, rather than in public schools that provide free education. In this way, the number of unaided private schools that provide paid education is expanding in India against the backdrop of rising national income.

However, despite this situation, public schools are more popular among prospective teachers than private schools. One of the reasons for this is that salaries in private

| | All area | Rural area |
|---|---|---|
| Primary only | **31.93** | **36.86** |
| Primary with upper primary | **24.88** | **24.84** |
| Primary with upper primary and secondary and higher secondary | 13.03 | 8.66 |
| Upper primary only | 6.93 | 8.55 |
| Upper primary with secondary and higher secondary | 8.13 | 7.57 |
| Primary with upper primary and secondary | 9.31 | 7.53 |
| Upper primary with secondary | 5.78 | 6.00 |
| All schools (N) | 8,323,024 | 6,108,966 |

**Table 5.**
*Percentage distribution of teachers by school category: 2016–2017.*

schools are not always paid, as stipulated by the government, and are not treated as well as teachers in public schools.

The survey data for the number of teachers in 2016–2017, as presented in the U-DISE, are shown in **Tables 5** and **6** [18].

An interview study with 29 Indian elementary school teachers revealed their views of classroom management (**Table 6**) [16]. The interview data were analyzed using a modified version of grounded theory, and 5 categories and 15 concepts were generated. The five categories identified are listed in **Table 7**.

### 4.1 Data collection and study participants

Teachers were selected based on the criterion of schools in four Indian states to which the authors had access. Twenty-nine teachers had elementary school experience. The quality level of teachers in Indian public schools was excluded because it was considered to vary widely, and most of the teachers were private school teachers. Three teachers from private Montessori schools were also included. Montessori schools are very popular in India. Only two of the public school teachers were trained by the American nonprofit foundation, Teachers for India: A Better Education Movement.

| | All government managements | All private managements |
|---|---|---|
| Primary only | 2.8 | **5.3** |
| Primary with upper primary | 6.4 | **8.5** |
| Primary with upper primary and secondary and higher secondary | 18.9 | **24.0** |
| Upper primary only | 3.7 | **4.9** |
| Upper primary with secondary and higher secondary | 23.0 | 15.9 |
| Primary with upper primary and secondary | 11.6 | **13.7** |
| Upper primary with secondary | 11.0 | 7.4 |
| All schools | 4.5 | **9.7** |

**Table 6.**
*Average number of teachers per school by school category: 2016–2017.*

| | Category | Definition |
|---|---|---|
| I | Clarify rules and responsibilities focus on teaching subjects | Teacher sets rules, develops a sense of responsibility in the child, and then concentrates on teaching the subject. |
| II | Respect for teachers while communicating between teachers and children | Teacher praises the child, communicates, and inculcates respect in the child for the teachers. |
| III | Frequent meetings with parents | There are frequent meetings with parents, and teachers and parents work together. |
| IV | Inclusive education and separation education | Inclusive education and separation education, and public schools that accept the poor. |
| V | Montessori education that stimulates children's senses | Performing Montessori education that stimulates children's senses. |

**Table 7.**
*Categories of classroom management for Indian elementary school teachers.*

### 4.2 Data collection period

The data collection period was from June to October 2018. Thus, the data collected were unaffected by the COVID-19 pandemic.

In Indian classroom management, the focus is team education. Elementary school teachers do not work alone but collaborate with many other professionals, such as assistant teachers, counselors, and school doctors.

There is a division of labor, with nonteaching staff providing instruction during nonclass hours such as recess, lunch, and special activities.

As mentioned earlier, many Indian elementary school teachers are in their 20s and 30s and have little experience; however, team education through multidisciplinary cooperation compensates for this lack of experience.

Elementary school teachers in India focus on the individuality of children to increase their motivation to learn and provide academic education. However, they did not have the perspective of a classroom group. The interviewee said, "There is a 45-minute lunch break, when the teacher returns to the staff room. Teachers are responsible for teaching the subjects and leave the school daily at 4 pm."

## 5. A comparison of Japanese and Indian classroom management

According to a 2018 UNICEF study, 59 million children of primary school did not go to school (**Table 8**). This represents 8 percent of children of that age. By region, 32 million children are in Africa, South of the Sahara, followed by 13 million in South Asia. Classroom management is one of the most important issues in the field of educational development and is a research field that aims to expand and improve educational opportunities.

However, it should be noted that classroom management as used in this educational development is the management of the "learning environment" to expand and improve educational opportunities, which is different in meaning from the "classroom management" used in Japan [19].

In Japan, classroom management is expected to play a broad role, not only in nurturing academic skills but also in developing children's personalities and socializing. However, in many Asian countries, the role of classroom management is to

| **Japanese-style classroom management** | | **Indian-style classroom management** |
|---|---|---|
| I Understanding children and connecting with children | Teacher's attitude toward children | II Respect for the teachers while communicating between teachers and children |
| V To develop into a chief through work | | |
| VI A teacher's attitude to learn from failure | | |
| III The will and skills of the homeroom teacher to give direction to the class while also providing special needs education | Teacher instruction and inclusive education | I Clarify rules and responsibilities focus on teaching subjects |
| | | IV Inclusive education and separation education |
| | | V Montessori education that stimulates children's senses |
| IV Responding to parents on the basis of responding to children | Cooperation with families | III Frequent meetings with parents |
| II Understanding the developmental stages of children and dealing with individuals and groups | Group activities | |

**Table 8.**
*Comparison of Japanese classroom management and Indian classroom management.*

provide the highest quality of education to as many children as possible. The Indian elementary schools that we compared in this study were in urban areas and attended by children from relatively affluent families. Therefore, while Indian elementary school teachers pay a lot of attention to teaching the subjects ("Teacher instruction and inclusive education"), they also value communication with children ("Teachers' attitude toward children") and do not miss cooperation with parents ("Cooperation with families"), similar to Japanese elementary school teachers.

On the other hand, the inclination toward "group activities" was not found among Indian elementary school teachers. According to Ishikawa, in Japanese school education, both academic and extracurricular activities are often conducted in the classroom. In addition, instruction in daily life, such as school lunches and cleaning, is conducted mainly in the classroom. Classroom management in Japan is not limited to classroom management for learning but extends to most school activities. Indian schools excel in terms of education toward multicultural understanding, and globalization. Therefore, it is necessary to clarify the actual classroom management situation of teachers in both the countries [20].

## 6. The Japanese style of classroom management that leads to long working hours

The reason for the long working hours of Japanese elementary school teachers lies in the Japanese-style classroom management.

**Figure 1** summarizes the overall picture of educational activities in Japanese elementary and junior high schools. School life in elementary and junior high schools generally lasts approximately 8 hours, from 8:00 a.m. to 4:00 p.m. (club activities in junior high schools are held until around 6:00 p.m.). The remaining two-fifths of the time is spent on nonacademic activities such as recess, cleaning, lunch, and after-school

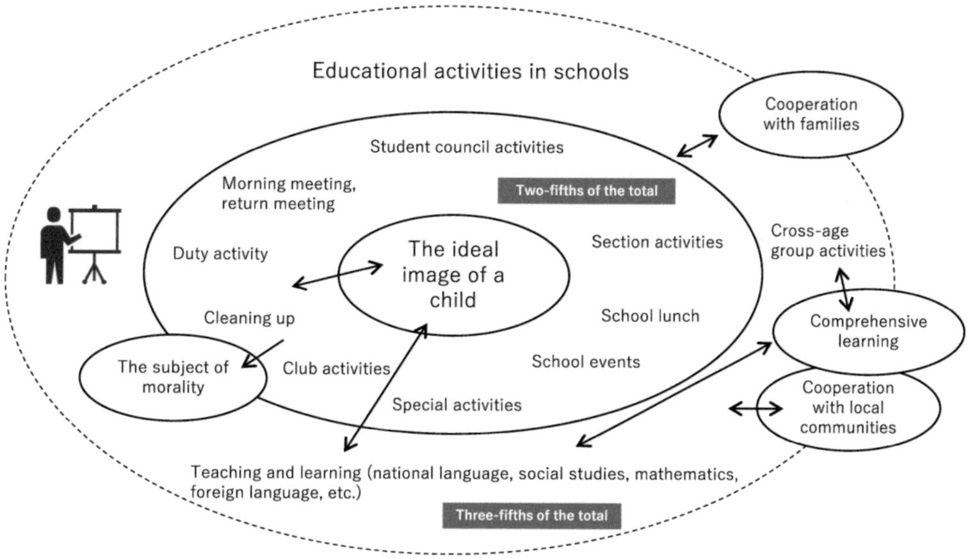


**Figure 1.**
*Overall concept of educational activities in schools.*

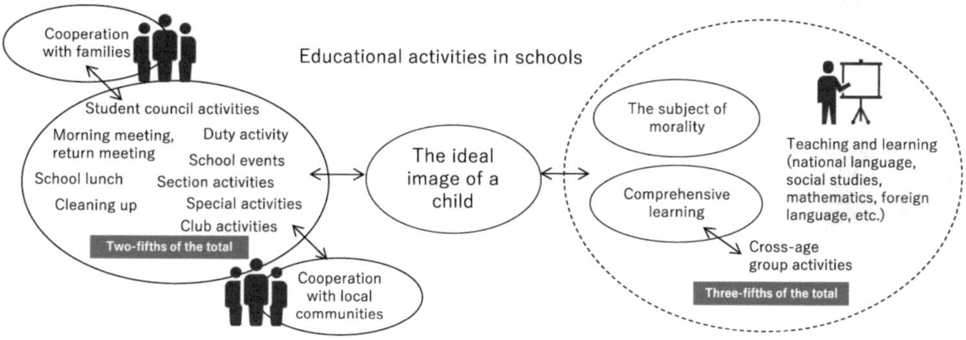


**Figure 2.**
*Shared Leadership in School Activities.*

activities. Surprisingly, in Japan, the classroom teacher plays the role of a leader not only during academic time but also during nonacademic times (**Figure 2**) [21].

## 7. New classroom management based on a mix model of Japanese classroom management

As we have seen, the long working hours of Japanese teachers, especially elementary school teachers, have resulted in work-related mental health issues, such as depression and adjustment disorders. The cause of the long working hours is Japanese-style classroom management.

Japanese education, which aims to build groups in the classroom while addressing the individual needs of children, strongly promotes not only academic learning but also the personal growth of children. In this sense, efforts to create groups in the classroom are unique.

The Japanese educational style has been introduced, and some countries have adopted it as a mixed model in their education system. In recent years, more and more schools in Egypt have introduced Japanese-style education, such as "special activities" (tokkatsu) [22]. However, it would be difficult to introduce such activities only by classroom teachers, as has been done in Japan.

Extracurricular activities are group-building activities. This activity should be incorporated into classroom management, but it is believed that multiple staff members are needed to carry out this activity. To achieve this, it is necessary to shift the leadership structure of teachers in schools from occupied to shared type. Discussions on reforming the leadership structure of teachers are also taking place in the United Kingdom and Canada [19].

Until now, teaching in Japan has been structured in such a way that the classroom teacher has a strong authority to guide the children, which is called "instructional leadership." When discussing the leadership of teachers, especially principals, there is an argument that we should move from instructional to shared leadership. In Japan, the leadership of the classroom teacher toward children is strong. Due to the extent of classroom management, a single classroom teacher tends to work too many hours. Therefore, a structure in which various people involved in the classroom perform the function of a leader based on the content of the activities seems to be suitable. In the Japanese style of classroom management, especially in "group activities," people other than classroom teachers can serve as leaders (**Figure 2**).

There is considerable discussion on the importance of interpersonal relationships, especially between teachers and students, in classroom management [4, 23–25]. Effective teacher-student interpersonal relationships have been shown to enhance students' academic performance and inhibit problem behaviors [8]. Conversely, poor teacher-student interpersonal relationships have been shown to have a significant impact not only on students but also on the mental health of teachers [26]. The teacher-student relationship centered on "group activities" in the new classroom management presented here emphasizes two-way communication, in which teachers and students interact to understand each other, rather than the one-way communication of academic instruction, in which teachers teach students.

While this chapter does not deal directly with the interpersonal relationship between teacher and student, the relationship is an important factor in the new "classroom management" presented here. In the future, it will be necessary to detail the interpersonal relationships between teachers and students within classroom management. The possibilities of new classroom management shown here can be applied to classroom management not only in Japan and India but also in other countries as well.

## 8. Conclusions

This chapter compares the Japanese and Indian classroom management styles of elementary school teachers, who are often responsible for classroom management, and discusses why the Japanese style of classroom management leads to long working hours.

In Japan, the number of teachers taking leave due to mental illness has been increasing annually, which is very high, even by international standards. One reason for this is the long working hours due to the various tasks and workload placed on classroom teachers alone. These long working hours have increased the rate of absenteeism due to mental illness among Japanese teachers. Through a comparison of the classroom management of elementary school teachers in India, it became clear that one of the reasons for long working hours is the Japanese-style classroom management. The Japanese-style classroom management is an excellent system that not only improves academic performance but also promotes children's personal growth. However, it is essential to reform the leadership structure of teachers when adopting this system.

Before introducing Japanese-style education to the international community, it is necessary to clarify its characteristics.

## Acknowledgements

This work was supported by JSPS KAKENHI (grant number 21 K02477). We would like to thank Editage (www.editage.com) for English language editing.

## Conflict of interest

The authors declare no conflict of interest.

## A. Appendices

a. Japanese Classroom Management Scale Items for Elementary School Teachers in Japan.

1. Creating a classroom with directions for dealing with the individual students and the group.

    - Whenever I have something good to say about a student, I try to speak comfortably with the child's parents promptly via phone calls and home visits.

    - I try to encourage the children to think about the classroom policies.

    - At class openings, I try to create an image for the students and their parents by showing the policies, strengths, and cheerfulness of the homeroom teacher. In the upper grades, I teach the students to form independent classroom groups.

    - In my dealings with parents, I emphasize that students should be at the center of the conversation.

    - For middle-grade students, I try to use their mischievous energy to help the group.

    - For students who need help, I created an individual chart and discussed ways to help them.

- Formulating and sharing rules, and reinforcing them with praise.
- Younger students who are not used to school life, we try to help them adjust to the group first.

2. Attitude as a teacher.

- I take pleasure with the changes in and growth of my students.
- I try to have a sincere attitude, sense of mission, and cheerfulness.
- I try to learn from my mistakes.
- I will make sure that I tell the students what they need to know and guide them properly.
- I try to grow so that I can become a head teacher in a few years.

3. Understanding individual children.

- Trying to understand each student's personality and life.
- Listening to students and interacting with them.
- Trying to notice the changes in each student's participation in different groups.

## Author details

Miyuki Matsumoto[1*], Michiko Ishikawa[2] and Sadananda Reddy[3]

1 Nagoya University, Nagoya, Japan

2 Nagoya Sangyo University, Nagoya, Japan

3 Jindal School of Psychology and Counselling, O.P. Jindal Global University, Sonepat, Haryana, India

*Address all correspondence to: matsumoto@cshe.nagoya-u.ac.jp

## References

[1] Syed Nurulla JN. History of Education in India During British Period. London: Macmillan and Co; 1943

[2] Venkatanarayanan S. Tracing the genealogy of elementary education policy in India till independence. Vol. 3. issue. 4. SAGE Open; 2013. DOI: 10.1177/2158244013510302

[3] Nishioka K. Classroom management in post war Japan. In: Evertson CM, Weinstein C, editors. Handbook of classroom management: Research, practice, and contemporary issues. Mahwah: Lawrence Erlbaum Associates; 2006. pp. 1215-1238

[4] Marzano RJ, Marzano JS. The Key to Classroom Management. Educational Leadership. 2003;**61**(1): 6-13

[5] Emmer ET, Stough LM. Classroom Management: A Critical Part of Educational Psychology, With Implications for Teacher Education. Educational Psychologist. 2001;**36**(2): 103-112

[6] Doyle W. Classroom organization and management. In: Wittrock M, editor. Handbook of Research on Teaching. 3rd ed. New York: Macmillan; 1986. pp. 392-431

[7] Brophy J. History of research on classroom management. In: Evertson CM, Weinstein CS, editors. Handbook of Classroom Management: Research, Practice, and Contemporary Issues. Mahwah, NJ: Lawrence Erlbaum Associates; 2006. pp. 17-43

[8] Evertson CM, Weinstein CS, Landrum TJ, Kauffman JM. Handbook of Classroom Management Research, Practice, and Contemporary Issues. New York: Routledge; 2013

[9] Ministry of Education, Culture, Sports, Science and Technology. Personnel Administration Status Survey of Public School Teachers in 2020, Tokyo. 2021. (In Japanese)

[10] Sogawa H. Improving the Mental Health of School Staff. Ministry of Education, Culture, Sports, Science and Technology, Document 2. 2018. pp. 1-41. (In Japanese)

[11] Senoo M. Teacher Collapse. Tokyo: PHP Institution; 2020. (In Japanese)

[12] Senoo M. Teacher and School Failure Studies. Tokyo: PHP Institution; 2021. (In Japanese)

[13] National Instutute for Educational Policy Research. International Comparison of Teacher Environments: Report of the OECD Teaching and Learning International Survey (TALIS) 2018- Teachers and Principals Continuing to Learn. Tokyo: Akashishoten; 2019. (In Japanese)

[14] Ishikawa M, Matsumoto M. Development of the Japanese Classroom Management Scale and Examination of its Reliability and Validity-Compared with Elementary School Teachers and Pre-Service Teachers. Tokoha University Faculty Education Research Bulletin. 2018;**4**:111-117

[15] Ishikawa M, Matsumoto M. What do Elementary School Teachers Think about a Teaching Classroom management?: Qualitative Analysis with the Modified Version Grounded Theory Approach. Tokoha University Faculty Education Research Bulletin. 2018;**4**: 17-27

[16] Ishikawa M, Odagiri M, Nakamura K, Matsumoto M. Indian Classroom Management among Elementary School Teachers in India. International Journal of Asia Pacific School of Psychology. 2020;**1**(2):139-153

[17] Ohara Y. Study on Unrecognized Schools in India: Shadow Institution's Supporting Public Education. Tokyo: Toshindo; 2014. (In Japanese)

[18] National Institute of Educational Planning and Administration. Analytical Tables 2016–17 Elementary Education in India. New Delhi: NIEPA; 2019

[19] Suematsu H, Hayashi K. Toward a Future of Classroom Management: Reality, Spirit and Hope. Tokyo: Gakubunsha; 2016

[20] Ishikawa M, Matsumoto M, Ramalingam P, Kamal M. Impact of Educational Guidance of Inclusive Education in Regular Classes and on Teacher Efficacy in India and Japan. International Journal of Asia Pacific School Psychology. 2022;**3**: 84-94

[21] Kitamura F. Classroom Management Reader. Tokyo: Tamagawa University Press; 2012. (In Japanese)

[22] Sawaji O. Tokkatsu Taking Root in Egypt. Public Relations Office, Government of Japan; 2019. Available from: https://www.gov-online.go.jp/eng/publicity/book/hlj/html/201907/201907_04_en.html. (Acceced date: 01/08/2022)

[23] Wubbels T. Brok PJ, Tartwijk JWF, Levy J. (Eds.) Interpersonal Relationships in Education: an Overview of Contemporary Research, (Advances in data mining and database management (ADMDM) book series). Sense Publishers; 2012. DOI: 10.1007/978-94-6091-939-8

[24] Wubbels T. An international perspective on classroom management: What should prospective teachers learn? Teaching Education. 2011;**22**(February): 113-131

[25] Wubbels T, Brekelmans M, den Brok P, van Tartwijk J. An interpersonal perspective on classroom management in secondary classrooms in The Netherlands. In: Handbook of Classroom Management. Routledge, The Netherlands; 2015. pp. 1171-1202

[26] Spilt JL, Koomen HMY, Thijs JT. Teacher wellbeing: The importance of teacher-student relationships. Educational Psychology Review. 2011; **23**(4):457-477

Chapter 3

# The Potential Role of Exercise-Induced Neurotrophic Factors for Mental Health

*Yakup Zühtü Birinci*

*"Ambulo ergo sum (I walk, therefore I am)" — Pierre Gassendi*

## Abstract

Today, there is a great scientific interest in understanding the mechanisms of mental disorders. Three lifestyle factors may play an essential role in protecting brain health: a socially integrated network, cognitive leisure activity, and regular exercise. It is widely accepted that exercise is a non-pharmacological, low-cost, easily accessible, and non-adverse promising method to delay brain deterioration in aging, and it was also suggested that exercise improves brain health across the lifespan. Despite the clear relationship between exercise and mental health, our knowledge of the cellular and molecular mechanisms that trigger such benefits is still limited. Pioneering studies showed that various peripheral factors (brain-derived neurotrophic factors, insulin-like growth factor-1, irisin, etc.) are released into the bloodstream via exercise. Moreover, there is much evidence that enhancement of neurogenesis, angiogenesis, and synaptogenesis caused by exercise-induced neurotrophins and growth factors, such as the BDNF, IGF-1, irisin, and VEGF, etc., has an essential role in the positive changes of mental health. Nevertheless, there is currently insufficient evidence to draw firm conclusions regarding the relationship between optimum exercise regime and maximize mental health via modulation of neurotrophic factors.

**Keywords:** BDNF, exercise, IGF-1, VEGF, Irisin, mental health

## 1. Introduction

Substantial evidence is that sedentary behavior associated with the so-called modern lifestyle increases the risk of obesity, cardiovascular disease, type 2 diabetes, osteoporosis, cancer, and depression. However, it is commonly thought that increasing the level of physical activity (PA) plays an essential role in preventing, reducing, managing, and treating these diseases with a wide variety of pathologies [1]. Although an active lifestyle has always been accepted as the best way to achieve health throughout civilization's history, since Hippocrates prescribed exercise for the first time in a patient, the concept of exercise as a medicine or a preventive method has been increasingly accepted in the last two decades [2–4]. Current studies report that exercise has a "polypill" feature with very low cost, no adverse effects, and nonpharmacological and easily accessible advantages compared to drugs, surgery, and hospitalization [5, 6].

The literature on the beneficial effects of exercise on health has generally focused on cardiovascular outcomes. However, studies pointed out that regular exercise can improve mental and physical health [7, 8]. According to Kramer [9], exercise acts like a drug with many beneficial effects. It should be prescribed not only for physical but also for mental health [9]. Several clinical studies [10–12] reported that exercise might trigger positive effects on different mental diseases, e.g., major depressive disorders (MDD), Alzheimer's dementia, and schizophrenia (SZ). While exercise facilitates adaptations to individuals' stress response systems, it can also improve physiological impairments imposed by psychological stressors [13]. Indeed, high levels of PA have been shown to reduce the risk of depression [14] and anxiety [15]. Many studies have shown that exercise can offer benefits comparable to antidepressant drugs in patients with depression [10, 16]. Similarly, current studies show that moderate to high-intensity daily exercises positively affect mental health, adversely affected by social isolation due to the pandemic [17].

The central questions that remain to be answered are whether or how exercise-induced neurotrophic factors impact mental health. Although many studies' results from the last decades have improved our understanding of the highly complex neurobiological and cognitive underlying mechanisms of mental health induced by exercise, many gray areas remain to be answered [18]. The putative idea that exercise can affect cognitive and behavioral functions positively has been extensively studied since the study of Van Praag et al., [19] allowing us to obtain cumulative information [19]. The pioneering study of Dishman et al. [20] showed for the first time that the prevention and treatment of diseases (including mental disorders) could be achieved through exercise-induced neurobiological mechanisms [20]. Today, exercise is thought to benefit mental health by mediating biochemical and physiological changes such as increased neurogenesis and decreased inflammatory and oxidant markers [21]. It is widely accepted that exercise, depending on the type, duration, and frequency, can trigger such benefits by increasing the levels of neuroprotective factors such as BDNF, irisin, vascular endothelial growth factor (VEGF), and insulin-like growth factor-1 (IGF-1) in the circulation or brain [22–24].

The relationship between the levels of these molecules (especially in the blood) and postexercise brain function may help identify biomarkers that can serve as objective indicators for clinically evaluating exercise therapy in the diseased or particularly aging brain. In addition, a better understanding of biomarkers may be instrumental in elucidating the mechanisms that mediate exercise-induced mental health. Thus, it can contribute to the discovery of new drugs or the creation of more effective exercise prescriptions for treatments to protect mental health. Due to the heterogeneous effect of exercise (exercise variables or levels of physical fitness and health status of person), it is, unfortunately, difficult to individualize an exercise regimen with optimal effects on mental health. Therefore, more research is needed to maximize the benefits of exercise to counter mental illness. Considering that there is currently no pharmaceutical drug or invasive method to treat neurodegenerative diseases, it will be important to evaluate the powerful potential of exercise to cope with neurodegenerative diseases [25].

In this regard, this paper aimed to summarize recent findings on candidate neurotrophic factors linked with mental health that exercise affects. It also focuses on identifying which exercise regime is an essential mediator of mental health and discuss whether there could be a generalized exercise prescription for optimizing mental health.

## 2. The potential role of exercise-induced neurotrophic factors on mental health

It is well reported that the potential role of exercise in providing or maintaining beneficial effects on mental health and inhibiting the disorder's progression is apparent. However, studies show that differences in the therapeutic benefit of exercise appear to be due to variations between populations and exercise modalities. The present literature suggests exercise-induced mental health with three mechanistic hypotheses; a) physical/hedonic effects, (b) neurobiological mechanisms, or (c) cultivating behavioral mechanisms of change. It seems that exercise simultaneously influences mental health via neurobiological and behavioral mechanisms [1]. However, this chapter focuses only on neurobiological mechanisms. Because the underlying mechanisms responsible for these beneficial effects are poorly defined, although some myokines and metabolites released by the skeletal muscle are well known to affect brain health positively, the underlying mechanisms require further investigation. This section will examine how different exercise protocols affect these mechanisms and the relationship of this effect with mental health.

### 2.1 Brain-derived neurotrophic factor (BDNF)

BDNF stands out due to its active role in the neurogenesis and neuroplasticity of neurons, which has a potential role in the pathophysiology of many neuropsychiatric disorders in various brain regions [26]. The cumulative evidence is diverse, including major depression [27, 28] bipolar disorder [29–31], and schizophrenia [32–34] shows that BDNF levels are significantly reduced in neuropsychiatric disorders. In addition, it has been shown that a decrease in hippocampal BDNF levels is associated with stress-induced depressive behaviors, and antidepressant treatment increases BDNF expression [35].

In addition, it is thought that BDNF may have different roles in brain stress and reward systems [36, 37]. Previous research showed that stress could change BDNF expression in many critical brain regions [38]. Underpin of this idea comes that BDNF and stressors can affect both systems: the stress-related system, which mainly contains the hypothalamus-pituitary–adrenocortical (HPA) axis and the hippocampus, and the reward-associated system, which mainly contains the ventral tegmental area–nucleus accumbens pathway [39]. BDNF may exert notable influences on these two systems. BDNF is also closely associated with insomnia, which is known to cause stress-related mental disorders [40]. Furthermore, limited studies have shown that direct hippocampal infusions of BDNF can produce antidepressant effects in rodents [41, 42]. Few human studies show that depressed patients have much lower BDNF levels in postmortem brain tissue than healthy human subjects [43]. It is hypothesized that low BDNF levels in the brain may cause atrophy and increased cell loss in the hippocampus and prefrontal cortex, as observed in depressed subjects [35, 44]. Similarly, most studies show decreased BDNF levels in schizophrenia [45]. Exercise benefits panic disorder (type of anxiety disorder) by increasing serum BDNF concentration [46].

It is well accepted that BDNF is the most sensitive neurotrophin to the effects of exercise [47]. Kurdi and Flora [48] investigated the role of aerobic exercise (AE) in affecting BDNF levels in the elderly with depression. Thirty-five older women (age $\geq$ 50 y) with depression and 35 healthy coeval women underwent treadmill running/walking with a speed of 6 km/h for 15 minutes once a day for 28 days. Before the intervention, the depression group's BDNF levels were far lower than in the non-depression group. Although AE increased BDNF production in both groups, the increasing percentage of BDNF levels was higher in the depression group. But important to note that subjects with depression were first treated with an antidepressant of selective serotonin reuptake inhibitors for 3 months before the intervention. A single-blind, randomized clinical trial design study compared standard psychiatric treatment and a 12-week AE program (60 min/3d/w, 10-min warm-up, followed by 45-min AE, and ended with a 5-min cool-down, 60–75% of $HR_{max}$) utilizing exergame (whole-body exercise software) and traditional AE equipment (a stationary bike, and an elliptical machine) in 33 individuals with schizophrenia [49]. The results indicate that AE is effective in enhancing neurocognitive functioning by BDNF up-regulation. Another found that a single exercise session (an incremental exercise test on a motorized treadmill) leads to a significant up-regulation and transient normalization of BDNF serum levels in elderly women (n = 35, age: 61.1 ± 7.2 y) with a remitted depressive episode of unipolar depression [50]. Kerling et al. [51] investigated the effect of 6 weeks AE (total 22 exercises, each exercise 45-min at moderate intensity, bicycle ergometer, treadmill, cross-trainer, and rowing) intervention on serum BDNF levels in guideline-based treated patients with MDD (n = 42, age: 44.2 ± 8.5 y). Authors indicated that AE given as an adjunct to standard guideline-based treatment has additional effects on serum BDNF levels in people with MDD. Moreover, Yeh et al. [52] observed that significant impact on the enhancement of BDNF levels and improvement of depression symptoms after 12 weeks AE (50-min/3d/w), with music in community women (n = 41, age: 53.2 ± 10.3 y).

A study by Hartmann et al. [53] revealed that 6 weeks of moderate-intensity AE (stationary cycling at 65% HRR for 35 min progressing to 70% for 40 min) reduces the severity of depression, anxiety, and psychological distress in people (age = 40.5 ± 9.84 y, n = 13) with mental health disorder compared to healthy counterparts. However, no difference was found between BDNF levels in the comparison between groups, and it was reported that there was no relationship between the effects of BDNF levels on disease symptoms. A randomized controlled study by Pereira et al. [54] investigated muscle strength exercises (hip flexion, abduction, adduction, and extension; knee flexion and extension; and mini-squat, 75% of 1RM) and AE (65%–80% of the $HR_{max}$, walking and calisthenics exercises) on the plasma levels of BDNF and depressive symptoms in 451 elderly women (community-dwelling older women, age: 65–89 y). Both protocols lasted 10 weeks, and 30 sessions (1-h sessions) in total were performed three times a week. Based on the findings, resistance exercise (RE) and AE improved depressive symptoms. Only SE significantly increased the plasma levels of BDNF. However, the authors indicated that BDNF did not mediate the positive effects of exercise on depressive symptoms in the elderly.

According to Birinci et al. [55], exergames, also known as active video games, are a new-generation exercise that can combine physical exercise and cognitive exercise at the same time. A randomized clinical trial by Anderson-Hanley et al. [56] investigated the effect of the cognitive benefit of exergame intervention and cognitive exercise in older adults (n = 14, age: 78.1 ± 9.9 y) with or at risk for mild cognitive impairment (MCI). Participants performed one of three conditions for 6 months:

exer-tour (low cognitive load, virtual scenic bike tour) or exer-score (high cognitive demand, videogame+biking or video game-only, no physical exercise). Exercises were conducted for at least 20 minutes at least twice a week and gradually increased exercise duration to 45 minutes and frequency to at least three to five times per week. Both exercise interventions had similarly positive effects on executive functions (Stroop and word memory test scores) after 6 months. In addition, increased BDNF level due to exercise was associated with increased gray matter volume in the prefrontal cortex and right anterior cingulate cortex. Byun and Kang [57] conducted aerobic and cognitive exercise separately in one session (50 min/4d/w, moderate-high intensity, cognitive exercise + AE, respectively) for 12 weeks in 24 women (age: 65–79 y). The cognitive exercise consisted of situation assessment, responding to language instruction, communication, counting with hand, drawing with hands, and following hand signals. The physical exercise included walking, stepping, knee up, leg up, hopping, jumping jack, squatting, lifting the heels, turning the leg, raising the arm, bending the wrist, and balancing exercises. Findings showed that the exercise program significantly increased the Mini-mental state examination scores and BDNF levels. Kim et al. [58] investigated the effect of a combined exercise [3d/w, RE: chest press, seated row, squat, shoulder press, biceps curl, triceps extension, calf raise, and reverse crunch with elastic band for 25 min, 12–13 RPE, and AE: moderate walking at 50−70% of heart rate reserve (HRR) for 25 min] program on circulating BDNF expression in 24 patients with schizophrenia for 12 weeks. Increased serum BDNF levels were observed following the combined exercise program. The authors pointed out that exercise-induced BDNF levels may provide an alternative treatment for the chronic schizophrenic population.

On the contrary, a randomized controlled trial by McGurk et al. [59] investigated the effect of adding a 30-h AE program over 10 weeks to an equally intensive cognitive remediation program on cognitive function. The study results showed a combination of physical exercise (stationary cycling, walking, or jogging 60–75% of $HR_{max}$, 3d/w/40 min) and cognitive exercise (computer-based games, 60 min/3d/w), and cognitive exercise alone improved cognitive functions. In addition, although there was no difference in BDNF levels between the groups, it was reported that moderate-intensity AE did not affect BDNF levels in people with mental disorders.

Some studies have also evaluated the effectiveness of a combination of exercise and behavioral therapy. Gourgouvelis et al. [60] recruited 16 individuals (4 M/12 F; age: 39.31 ± 1.25 y) with MDD or anxiety and 22 healthy individuals (11 M/11 F; age: 20.95 ± 1.25 y) in their study. The authors investigated the effects of exercise on treatment outcomes in addition to antidepressant medication and behavioral therapy for 8 weeks. Exercise with behavioral therapy was conducted for 8 weeks [≥150 min/w AE at 60–80% $HR_{max}$ and 2d/w RE (8–12 repetitions at 95% of 10 repeated maximum, 2–3 superset large muscle groups]. After the intervention, 75% of patients showed either a therapeutic response or a complete remission of symptoms, resulting in a greater reduction in depression symptoms compared to 25% of non-exercise. In a study by Szuhany and Otto [61], participants with MDD or dysthymia (n = 29, 22 F/7 M, age: 18–65 y) performed 16 weeks of behavioral therapy (experts performed individual interview, 60 min/3d/w) or behavioral therapy+exercise (150 min/w moderate-intensity AE or mild-intensity yoga) or behavioral therapy+stretching (150 min/w) intervention. BDNF is increased in the depressive sedentary population immediately after acute exercise. Although acute exercise has increased BDNF levels in depressed individuals, no correlation was found between BDNF changes and changes in depression symptoms. Ikai et al. [62] investigated the effects of Hatha yoga therapy on resilience and BDNF levels activity in patients with schizophrenia-spectrum disorders. While the yoga group performed weekly 1-hour Hatha yoga sessions [gentle yoga stretches and simple movements in coordination with breathing, movements of major muscle groups, asana (twisting poses and standing poses), deep relaxation, and breathing exercises] in addition to regular treatment, the control group recruited a daycare rehabilitation program (provided social skills and walking). No significant differences were found in changes in BDNF levels from baseline to week eight between the two groups. The authors also indicated that yoga therapy showed no beneficial effects on the resilience level of stress markers.

According to Szuhany and Otto [61], effect sizes indicate that studies with approximately 85 participants may be needed to obtain significant associations between BDNF response and depression outcome in cases where exercise is not the only treatment method. Furthermore, as previous studies have shown that BDNF responds differently to the gender variant, obtaining comparable samples of men and women may be essential to assess its effects [24, 63]. Studies generally evaluate 150 minutes of moderate-intensity exercise per week. However, the current literature reports that short-term high-intensity interval training (HIIT) would increase BDNF levels significantly [64, 65]. Therefore, future studies can add the HIIT method to exercise programs to get a clearer understanding of the exercise effect. In addition, it should consider that some drugs used by participants under treatment may create confusion when revealing the effect of exercise alone. Moreover, results from sample groups with wide age ranges may influence the inferences because it is well known that BDNF levels are affected by age [66].

### 2.2 Irisin

Inducing peroxisome proliferator-activated receptor-gamma coactivator-1 alpha (PGC-1$\alpha$) by exercise leads to the production of the muscle protein called fibronectin type III domain containing 5 (FNDC5). Then FNDC5 cleaved and generates a polypeptide hormone named irisin. Irisin is a recently discovered exercise-induced myokine that can control numerous cellular signaling (white fat-browning, energy expenditure increase, anti-inflammatory effects, and mitochondrial function improvement) in many organs [67]. Irisin is expressed in skeletal muscles [68], adipose tissue, pancreas, cardiac muscle [69], and several regions of the brain [70, 71] and is also observed in Purkinje cells, neurons in the cerebellum [71], and cerebrospinal fluid [72]. Moreover, a large number of investigations reported that RE (eight exercises of 12 repetitions with 3–4 sets at 65% of 1RM) [73], prolonged moderate AE (a 90-min treadmill exercise protocol at 60% of $VO2_{max}$) [74], and strenuous exercise (a 30-min cycling ergometry) [75] induce the peripheral irisin levels. Jedrychowski et al. demonstrated that irisin circulates at ~3.6 ng/ml in sedentary individuals, while it can significantly increase in individuals undergoing AE up to ~4.3 ng/ml [76].

Irisin may have an impact on the expression of many neuronal genes that modulate neuronal plasticity [77, 78] and that can potentially fight against neural deterioration [79] and are secreted strongly by exercise [68, 77]. Some studies also suggest that irisin is likely to have a beneficial effect hippocampus and dentate gyrus, which are memory-related brain regions [80, 81]. A review study by Farshbaf and Alvina, [67] indicated that irisin has multiple endocrine actions central nervous system and this molecular mechanism can show neuroprotection against different injuries and insults, including neurodegenerative disorders. Authors also pointed out that irisin release can modulate BDNF expression in the hippocampus leading to protection against ischemia, acute stress, and neurodegenerative disorders. They suggested that pharmacologically FNDC5/Irisin could be an alternative as mimetic of exercise, in cases for example that exercise is not recommended or not possible. In a pioneering study, Lourenco et al. [79] found that the expression of FNDC5 in the hippocampus and cerebrospinal fluid is decreased in both human and mouse models with AD. Similarly, decreased PGC-1α expression was observed in human Parkinson's disease (PD) brain samples [82]. Yu et al. [83] showed that cerebral ischemia can reduce FNDC5 expression in skeletal muscle and circulating irisin levels in the peripheral blood.

Recently, irisin is thought to be a therapeutic hormone that can positively affect depressive behaviors through its effect on neuronal activities in the prefrontal cortex [84, 85]. Moreover, some studies suggest that exercise-induced irisin ameliorates depressive symptoms by activating the PGC-1α-FNDC5/irisin pathway in the hippocampus [21, 86]. Irisin upregulates BDNF expression in many brain areas (VTA, hippocampus, etc.), involved in learning, mood, attention, motivation, and reward system. Irisin levels lead to improve mitochondria function through PGC-1α signaling and elevate BDNF enhancing synaptic plasticity in the brain. Finally, this process may lead to the improvement of depressive neuropathology (**Figure 1**). Similarly, Siteneski et al. [87] indicated that central administration of irisin and BDNF elicited antidepressant-like behaviors in mice. Studies also observed decreased serum irisin levels in people with post-stroke depression [88] and anxiety disorder [89].

Papp et al. [90] revealed that irisin might link mood deterioration to the central effects of BDNF exerted in areas closely associated with reward-related processes involved in the evolution of depression in patients with chronic obstructive pulmonary disease ($n = 74$, age: $62.15 \pm 9.70$ y). Similarly, Zsuga et al. [91] indicated that exercise-induced irisin might have a role in motivation and reward-related processes. Wrann et al. [77] revealed that the proliferation of FNDC5 in the primary cortical neurons may have increased expression of BDNF. A study investigating the relationship between energy homeostasis regulation and coronary heart disease (CHD) patients comorbid with depression by Han et al. [92] indicated that interaction between irisin and BDNF could trigger the imbalance of energy homeostasis in the depression of CHD patients. They also demonstrated that irisin and BDNF serum levels were significantly lower in CHD patients with depression compared with CHD patients without depression. Similarly, a review study by Jo and Song [93] suggests that irisin is an essential molecule that may suppress several neuropathological mechanisms involved in depression. On the contrary, Hofmann et al. [94] investigated the effectiveness of irisin release with depressiveness, perceived stress, and anxiety symptoms in obese women ($n = 98$, age: $43.9 \pm 12.5$ y). According to their study results, irisin was not associated with depressiveness, anxiety, and perceived stress in female obese patients.

### 2.3 Insulin-like growth factor-1 (IGF-1)

IGF-1 can modulate many mechanisms that help to occur neuroplasticity in the human brain, such as synaptic processes (e.g., long-term potentiation) [95, 96], angiogenesis, axon outgrowth, dendritic maturation, and synaptogenesis [97, 98]. Moreover, there is a putative idea that IGF-1 plays a role in structural gray matter changes. Supporting neuronal survival via inducing proliferation, reducing apoptosis, and protecting neurons against toxicity may underpin this idea [99]. According to Calvo et al. [100] higher levels of serum IGF-1 are associated with better cognitive

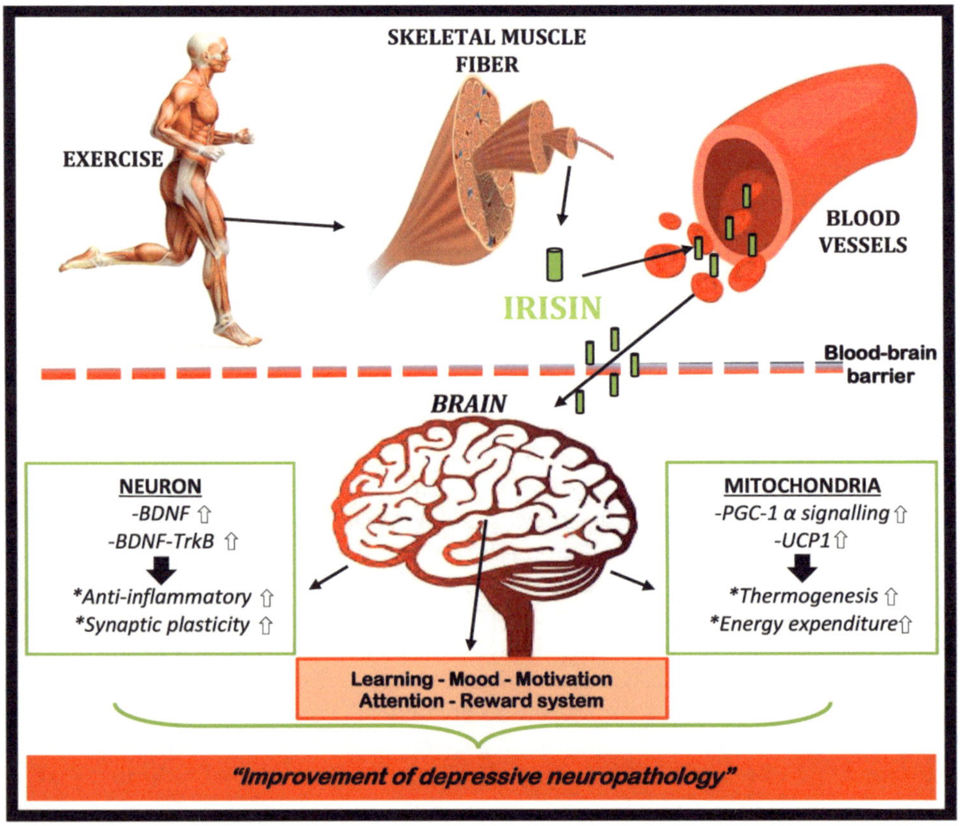


**Figure 1.**
*The effect of exercise on the irisin pathway and related depressive neuropathology changes. Exercise-induced irisin is mainly derived from skeletal muscle and readily crosses the blood–brain barrier. Irisin upregulates BDNF expression in many brain areas involved in learning, mood, attention, motivation, and reward system. Irisin levels lead to improve mitochondria function through PGC-1α signaling and elevate BDNF enhancing synaptic plasticity in the brain. Finally, this process may lead to the improvement of depressive neuropathology. FNDC5, fibronectin domain-containing protein 5; PGC-1α, proliferator-activated receptor-gamma coactivator-1 alpha; UCP1, uncoupling protein 1; BDNF, brain-derived neurotrophic factor; TrkB, tropomyosin receptor kinase B.*

performance in persons (n = 31, age: 83.71 ± 3.59 y, 58% women) with MCI, particularly on tests of learning and memory. A cross-sectional study by Duron et al. [101] showed a significant association between low IGF-I serum levels and neurodegenerative process of AD in men, but not in women (218 men, 476 women; 78.6 ± 6.7 y). Parallel to this, evidence suggests that IGF-1 may have a role in beta-amyloid clearance and reducing hyperphosphorylation tau in AD [102].

A recent review revealed that IGF-1 serum levels might be affected by the type of exercise. However, there is no consensus on the effect of exercise conditions yet [103]. A study by Cassilhas et al. [104] showed that 24 weeks of intensive RE (6 exercises: chest press, leg press, vertical traction, abdominal crunch, leg curl, and lower back, 80% of the 1RM, 2 sets of 8 repetitions each with rests for 1-min 30-sec between them and 3-min between exercises) intervention improved mood, ameliorated anxiety, and increased IGF-1 serum concentration in older men (n = 20) ages 65 to 75 years. Yoon et al. [105] recruited 30 older women into the RE and interval training group (n = 10, age: 64.10 ± 3.35 y), the RE and AE group (n = 10, age: 65.20 ± 5.10 y), and the control group (n = 10, age: 63.20 ± 2.62 y). Authors aimed to determine the effects of RE (chest press, lateral pull-down, arm curl, back extension, crunch, leg press, leg extension, leg curl, and heel raise, 8–15 repeat at the intensity of 1-RM, 60–80%, in 3 sets) + AE (stationary bicycle exercise for 30 mi at the target HR of 50–60%) and RE+ interval training (stationary bicycle exercise different durations at different HR, HR variability 40% between 90%) on the mental health in older women. Participants performed 12 weeks of exercise involving 30-minute RE followed by 30-min interval training or AE 3 times a week. Not depending on the type of exercise, both interventions effectively changed the IGF-1 levels, functional fitness, and sleep quality. However, no difference was found between the two types of exercise. A recent study investigated circulating IGF-1 levels in AD patients (n = 34) and older adults (n = 40) without dementia after acute exercise (Balke-Ware test: incremental test on a treadmill), [102]. After the intervention, higher levels of IGF-1 were observed in AD patients. Tsai et al. [106] investigated the effects of acute AE (a 30-minute bout of bicycle ergometer exercise at 65–75% of HRR) or RE (30-minute biceps curls, triceps extensions, bench presses, leg presses, leg extensions, and vertical butterflies exercises for two sets of 10 repetitions, at 75% 1RM, with a 90-second rest between sets, and a 2 minutes interval between each different exercise) interventions on neurocognitive performances and changes in circulating levels of neuroprotective growth factors (e.g., BDNF, IGF-1, and VEGF) in older adults (n = 55, age: 60–80 y) with amnestic MCI. Findings of the study showed that an acute bout of AE significantly increased serum levels of BDNF and IGF-1, but only serum IGF-1 levels increasing were observed after RE.

Ding et al. [107] indicated that IGF-1 also contributes to the BDNF pathway to mediate exercise-induced synaptic and cognitive plasticity. Thus, stimulation of the uptake of blood-borne IGF-I by nerve cells may lead to the synergetic neuroprotective effect by inducing BDNF levels [108]. Similarly, a review pointed out that there is a putative idea about the possible pharmacological and biochemical mechanisms of several types of antidepressants (selective serotonin reuptake inhibitors) and antipsychotics, in which activation of IGF-1 and BDNF pathways seem to drive the therapeutic effects [109]. Nevertheless, besides the IGF-1, mechanisms such as hormonal involvement, neurotransmitter levels, and the balance between sympathetic and parasympathetic central activity should also consider for the neurobiology of depression [104]. A recent review investigated the molecular mechanisms of exercise in the coronavirus disease 19 (COVID-19) pandemic on mental health [110]. It indicated that exercise enhances IGF-1 levels and the activity of the PGC-1α/FNDC5/Irisin pathway leading to neuronal survival and the maintenance of good mental health, which is poorly affected in the quarantine period during COVID-19.

### 2.4 Vascular endothelial growth factor (VEGF)

VEGF is a signal protein belonging to a subfamily of growth factors. It is produced by cells that stimulate the formation of blood vessels [111]. VEGF is classically associated with stimulation of angiogenesis and vasculogenesis [112]. However, recent evidence has shown that it also affects nerve cells and plays an important role in hippocampal neurogenesis and neuroprotection [113]. As BDNF or IGF-1, exercise-induced VEGF may have a role in ameliorating the pathological process of AD [114]. Moreover, VEGF, because of its active role in neurogenesis, may mediate antidepressant therapies [115]. These authors revealed that VEGF level changes were not associated with depressive symptom improvement due to repetitive transcranial magnetic stimulation but strongly correlated with reduction of anhedonia. Another study showed higher serum VEGF levels in non-responders than in responder patients with MDD treated with antidepressants [116]. A recent study pointed out that VEGF is linked with increased BBB permeability [117]. It could be an important pathology linking stress and psychiatric disorders, including MDD. Results of the study indicated that VEGF might play an essential role in the pathogenesis of depression by increasing the BBB permeability. Parallel to these findings, Hadidi et al. [118] indicated various neurological and physical symptoms due to post-stroke depression (PSD), including a decrease in serum BDNF and VEGF levels A study revealed that VEGF-induced antidepressant-like effects involve modulation of norepinephrine and serotonin systems [119].

VEGF is a candidate anti-stress molecule because of its role in enhancing antidepressant-like effects in response to different external stimuli such as stress, learning and exercise [119]. An animal study showed that exercise can be leading the expression of VEGF, especially in the hippocampus [120]. In humans, an immediate increase was shown in serum VEGF levels after high-altitude exercise and its effect lasted up to 1 month after training [121]. On the contrary, another study indicate that exercise did not have a positive effect on VEGF [122].

Krogh et al. [123] investigated the effect of an AE (45 min/3d/w for 3 months, stationary bike at 80% of $HR_{max}$) intervention on hippocampal volume and serum BDNF, VEGF, and IGF-1 in patients with MDD (n = 79, age: 18–60 y). In conclusion, the authors observed no significant increase in resting levels of neurotrophins. But they pointed out a positive association between change in hippocampal volume and depressive symptoms. A randomized controlled trial revealed that in older adults (n = 55) with amnestic MCI, both exercise regimes (16 weeks) AE and RE are effective in increasing neurotrophins (BDNF, IGF-1, and VEGF, etc.,) reducing some inflammatory cytokines, and facilitating neurocognitive performance [124]. Another study [106] showed that VEGF levels tended to increase after AE but no significant changes were observed after RE. Du et al. [125] compared the acute effects of high (80% 1-RM) and low (40% 1-RM) RE (sitting pull-down, sitting shoulder press, sitting chest push, sitting leg kick) with or without blood flow restriction on perception, BDNF, and VEGF levels in patients (N = 24) with post-stroke depression (PSD). Based on the findings, there were no increases in BDNF and VEGF levels of each group compared to before exercise. After exercise, the BDNF levels of the low RE group increased significantly, but without change was observed in the VEGF level of the low RE group. In addition, blood flow restriction RE may increase the serum BNDF and VEGF levels of PSD patients by increasing the body's blood lactic acid concentration.

## 3. Conclusions

This paper summarizes the recent literature on the potential role of exercise-induced neurotrophic factors on mental health. This paper indicates that there is much evidence that the enhancement of neurogenesis, angiogenesis, and synaptogenesis caused by exercise-induced neurotrophins and growth factors, such as the BDNF, IGF-1, irisin, and VEGF, etc., has an essential role in the positive changes of mental health including depression, anxiety, cognition and psychosis. Nevertheless, there is currently insufficient evidence to draw firm conclusions regarding the relationship between optimum exercise regimes to maximize mental health via modulation of neurotrophic factors.

It is also important to note that there is a considerable gap in evidence [126] for the causative relationship between exercise, neurotrophic factors, and brain function and exercise's effect on neuropsychiatric function. Moreover, compared to BDNF, the most studied neurotrophic factor, there is still insufficient evidence for a clear explanation of the association between exercise and other candidates such as irisin, IGF-1, and VEGF levels or their-mediated exercise benefit on mental disorders. A mental disorder may have many symptoms affecting multiple neural processes [127]. The contradictory results from studies due to the wide variety of symptoms make it challenging to target a disorder itself- or symptoms-specific exercise prescription to optimize mental health.

On the other hand, although numerous previous studies reported the beneficial effect of exercise on mental health, it should consider that the effect level highly depends on the type, duration, frequency and intensity of the exercise regime. Exercise variables that provide different cognitive, metabolic, or physiological loads can cause different neurotrophic factors to be released [128]; therefore, the effects of different types of exercises on the neurochemical system and mental disorders may also be unique to them. Understanding the crosstalk between dynamic neurobiological factors and exercise variables (type, frequency, intensity, etc.,) may help optimize personalized mental health exercise programs.

While the studies examining the beneficial effects of exercise on mental health have focused on long-term adaptations, the acute beneficial effects of exercise mediated by peripheral neurotrophic factors are not well characterized. It must be taken into consideration that investigating acute responses to an exercise might help us to explain the underlying functional and molecular mechanisms of how long-term mental health adaptation occur. Due to the positive neurotrophic factor responses from different types of exercise, studies can be planned to evaluate whether multimodal exercise interventions which combine AE, RE or cognitive exercise methods can contribute a greater beneficial effect on mental health.

The social distancing and/or isolation period during the COVID-19 pandemic led greater prevalence of mental health disorders such as depression and anxiety [129]. Considering that the pandemic is not over yet and isolation obligations are possible in other diseases in the future, the planning of exercise programs such as exergame that people can apply at home will be important in maintaining mental health [130].

Lastly, considering that there is still no fully invasive or pharmacologically effective treatment for mental health, it makes sense to exploit the potential of exercise to produce beneficial effects on mental health through neurotrophic factors. Besides the fact that exercise can improve mental health, it can also provide other benefits such as improved quality of life, good sleep quality, increased muscle mass, and greater cardiovascular condition. These benefits will be far more inclusive than the current pharmacological treatments.

## Acknowledgements

I would like to thank all the precious scientists in the references section for their valuable contributions to the field.

## Conflict of interest

The authors declare no conflict of interest.

## Author details

Yakup Zühtü Birinci
Faculty of Sports Science, Bursa Uludag University, Bursa, Turkey

*Address all correspondence to: ykpbirinci@gmail.com

## References

[1] Smith PJ, Merwin RM. The role of exercise in management of mental health disorders: An integrative review. Annual Review of Medicine. 2012;**72**:45. DOI: 10.1146%2Fannurev-med-060619-022943

[2] Birinci YZ. Veteran sporcularda farklı tip akut egzersizin serum beyin kaynaklı nörotrofik faktör (BDNF) düzeyleri ve nörobilişsel işlevler üzerine etkisi [Doctoral thesis] Bursa Uludag University; 2021

[3] Sallis RE. Exercise is medicine and physicians need to prescribe it! British Journal of Sports Medicine. 2009;**43**(1):3-4. DOI: 10.1136/bjsm.2008.054825

[4] Tipton CM. The history of "exercise is medicine" in ancient civilizations. Advances in Physiology Education. 2014;**38**(2):109-117. DOI: 10.1152/advan.00136.2013

[5] Deslandes AC. Exercise and mental health: What did we learn in the last 20 years? Frontiers in Psychiatry. 2014;**5**:66. DOI: 10.3389/fpsyt.2014.00066

[6] Swenson S, Blum K, McLaughlin T, Gold MS, Thanos PK. The therapeutic potential of exercise for neuropsychiatric diseases: A review. Journal of the Neurological Sciences. 2020;**412**:116763. DOI: 10.1016/j.jns.2020.116763

[7] Albagmi FM, Alansari A, Al Shawan DS, AlNujaidi HY, Olatunji SO. Prediction of generalized anxiety levels during the Covid-19 pandemic: A machine learning-based modeling approach. Informatics in Medicine Unlocked. 2022;**28**:100854. DOI: 10.1016/j.imu.2022.100854

[8] Carmassi C, Dell'Osso L, Bertelloni CA, Pedrinelli V, Dell'Oste V, Cordone A, et al. Three-month follow-up study of mental health outcomes after a national COVID-19 lockdown: Comparing patients with mood or anxiety disorders living in an area with a higher versus lower infection incidence. The Journal of Clinical Psychiatry. 2022;**83**(2):39558

[9] Kramer A. An overview of the beneficial effects of exercise on health and performance. In: Junjie X, editor. Physical Exercise for Human Health. Singapore: Springer Nature; 2020. pp. 3-22. DOI: 10.1007/978-981-15-1792-1_1

[10] Blumenthal JA, Sherwood A, Rogers SD, Babyak MA, Murali Doraiswamy P, Watkins L, et al. Understanding prognostic benefits of exercise and antidepressant therapy for persons with depression and heart disease: The UPBEAT study—Rationale, design, and methodological issues. Clinical Trials. 2007;**4**(5):548-559. DOI: 10.1177%2F1740774507083388

[11] Hirsch MA, Toole T, Maitland CG, Rider RA. The effects of balance training and high-intensity resistance training on persons with idiopathic Parkinson's disease. Archives of Physical Medicine and Rehabilitation. 2003;**84**(8):1109-1117. DOI: 10.1016/S0003-9993(03)00046-7

[12] Rolland Y, Pillard F, Klapouszczak A, Reynish E, Thomas D, Andrieu S, et al. Exercise program for nursing home residents with Alzheimer's disease: A 1-year randomized, controlled trial. Journal of the American Geriatrics Society. 2007;**55**(2):158-165. DOI: 10.1111/j.1532-5415.2007.01035.x

[13] Sothmann MS, Buckworth J, Claytor RP, Cox RH, White-Welkley JE, Dishman RK. Exercise training and the cross-stressor adaptation hypothesis. Exercise and Sport Sciences Reviews. 1996;**24**(1):267-288

[14] Schuch FB, Vancampfort D, Firth J, Rosenbaum S, Ward PB, Silva ES, et al. Physical activity and incident depression: A meta-analysis of prospective cohort studies. American Journal of Psychiatry. 2018;**175**(7):631-648. DOI: 10.1176/appi.ajp.2018.17111194

[15] McDowell CP, Dishman RK, Gordon BR, Herring MP. Physical activity and anxiety: A systematic review and meta-analysis of prospective cohort studies. American Journal of Preventive Medicine. 2019;**57**(4):545-556. DOI: 10.1016/j.amepre.2019.05.012

[16] Blumenthal JA, Babyak MA, Moore KA, Craighead WE, Herman S, Khatri P, et al. Effects of exercise training on older patients with major depression. Archives of Internal Medicine. 1999;**159**(19):2349-2356. DOI: 10.1001/archinte.159.19.2349

[17] Jacob L, Tully MA, Barnett Y, Lopez-Sanchez GF, Butler L, Schuch F, et al. The relationship between physical activity and mental health in a sample of the UK public: A cross-sectional study during the implementation of COVID-19 social distancing measures. Mental Health and Physical Activity. 2020;**19**:100345. DOI: 10.1016/j.mhpa.2020.100345

[18] Gillan CM, Rutledge RB. Smartphones and the neuroscience of mental health. Annual Review of Neuroscience. 2021;**44**:129-151. DOI: 10.1146%2Fannurev-neuro-101220-014053

[19] Van Praag H, Kempermann G, Gage FH. Running increases cell proliferation and neurogenesis in the adult mouse dentate gyrus. Nature Neuroscience. 1999;**2**(3):266-270. DOI: 10.1038/6368

[20] Dishman RK, Berthoud HR, Booth FW, Cotman CW, Edgerton VR, Fleshner MR, et al. Neurobiology of exercise. Obesity. 2006;**14**(3):345-356. DOI: 10.1038/oby.2006.46

[21] Schuch FB, Deslandes AC, Stubbs B, Gosmann NP, da Silva CTB, de Almeida Fleck MP. Neurobiological effects of exercise on major depressive disorder: A systematic review. Neuroscience & Biobehavioral Reviews. 2016;**61**:1-11. DOI: 10.1016/j.neubiorev.2015.11.012

[22] Birinci YZ, Sagdilek E, Taymur I, Budak E, Beyaz A, Vatansever S, et al. Acute effects of different types of exercises on insulin-like growth factor-1, homocysteine and cortisol levels in veteran athletes. Medicine. 2022;**11**(3):968-974. DOI: 10.5455/medscience.2022.02.028

[23] Birinci YZ, Şahin Ş, Vatansever Ş, Pancar S. Yaşlılarda fiziksel egzersizin beyin kaynaklı nörotrofik faktör (bdnf) üzerine etkisi: deneysel çalışmaların sistematik derlemesi. Spor Hekimliği Dergisi. 2019;**54**(4):276-287. DOI: 10.5152/tjsm.2019.142

[24] Dinoff A, Herrmann N, Swardfager W, Lanctot KL. The effect of acute exercise on blood concentrations of brain-derived neurotrophic factor in healthy adults: A meta-analysis. European Journal of Neuroscience. 2017;**46**(1):1635-1646. DOI: 10.1111/ejn.13603

[25] Mahalakshmi B, Maurya N, Lee SD, Bharath Kumar V. Possible neuroprotective mechanisms of physical exercise in neurodegeneration. International Journal of Molecular

Sciences. 2020;**21**(16):5895. DOI: 10.3390/ijms21165895

[26] Nagahara AH, Tuszynski MH. Potential therapeutic uses of BDNF in neurological and psychiatric disorders. Nature Reviews Drug Discovery. 2011;**10**(3):209-219. DOI: 10.1038/nrd3366

[27] Molendijk ML, Spinhoven P, Polak M, Bus BAA, Penninx BWJH, Elzinga BM. Serum BDNF concentrations as peripheral manifestations of depression: Evidence from a systematic review and meta-analyses on 179 associations (N= 9484). Molecular Psychiatry. 2014;**19**(7):791-800. DOI: 10.1038/mp.2013.105

[28] Teche SP, Nuernberg GL, Sordi AO, de Souza LH, Remy L, Ceresér KMM, et al. Measurement methods of BDNF levels in major depression: A qualitative systematic review of clinical trials. Psychiatric Quarterly. 2013;**84**(4):485-497. DOI: 10.1007/s11126-013-9261-7

[29] Fernandes BS, Gama CS, Ceresér KM, Yatham LN, Fries GR, Colpo G, et al. Brain-derived neurotrophic factor as a state-marker of mood episodes in bipolar disorders: A systematic review and meta-regression analysis. Journal of Psychiatric Research. 2011;**45**(8):995-1004. DOI: 10.1016/j.jpsychires.2011.03.002

[30] Munkholm K, Vinberg M, Kessing LV. Peripheral blood brain-derived neurotrophic factor in bipolar disorder: A comprehensive systematic review and meta-analysis. Molecular Psychiatry. 2016;**21**(2):216-228. DOI: 10.1038/mp.2015.54

[31] Wang D, Li H, Du X, Zhou J, Yuan L, Ren H, et al. Circulating brain-derived neurotrophic factor, antioxidant enzymes activities, and mitochondrial DNA in bipolar disorder: An exploratory report. Frontiers in Psychiatry. 2020;**11**:514658. DOI: 10.3389%2Ffpsyt.2020.514658

[32] Fernandes BS, Steiner J, Berk M, Molendijk ML, Gonzalez-Pinto A, Turck CW, et al. Peripheral brain-derived neurotrophic factor in schizophrenia and the role of antipsychotics: meta-analysis and implications. Molecular Psychiatry. 2015;**20**(9):1108-1119. DOI: 10.1038/mp.2014.117

[33] Song X, Quan M, Lv L, Li X, Pang L, Kennedy D, et al. Decreased cortical thickness in drug naive first episode schizophrenia: in relation to serum levels of BDNF. Journal of Psychiatric Research. 2015;**60**:22-28. DOI: 10.1016/j.jpsychires.2014.09.009

[34] Sanada K, Zorrilla I, Iwata Y, Bermúdez-Ampudia C, Graff-Guerrero A, Martínez-Cengotitabengoa M, et al. The efficacy of non-pharmacological interventions on brain-derived neurotrophic factor in schizophrenia: A systematic review and meta-analysis. International Journal of Molecular Sciences. 2016;**17**(10):1766. DOI: 10.3390/ijms17101766

[35] Duman RS, Monteggia LM. A neurotrophic model for stress-related mood disorders. Biological Psychiatry. 2006;**59**(12):1116-1127. DOI: 10.1016/j.biopsych.2006.02.013

[36] Berton O, McClung CA, DiLeone RJ, Krishnan V, Renthal W, Russo SJ, et al. Essential role of BDNF in the mesolimbic dopamine pathway in social defeat stress. Science. 2006;**311**(5762):864-868. DOI: 10.1126/science.1120972

[37] Eisch AJ, Bolaños CA, De Wit J, Simonak RD, Pudiak CM, Barrot M, et al. Brain-derived neurotrophic factor in the ventral midbrain–nucleus accumbens pathway: A role in depression. Biological

Psychiatry. 2003;**54**(10):994-1005. DOI: 10.1016/j.biopsych.2003.08.003

[38] Chattarji S, Tomar A, Suvrathan A, Ghosh S, Rahman MM. Neighborhood matters: Divergent patterns of stress-induced plasticity across the brain. Nature Neuroscience. 2015;**18**(10):1364-1375. DOI: 10.1038/nn.4115

[39] Miao Z, Wang Y, Sun Z. The relationships between stress, mental disorders, and epigenetic regulation of BDNF. International Journal of Molecular Sciences. 2020;**21**(4):1375. DOI: 10.3390/ijms21041375

[40] Schmitt K, Holsboer-Trachsler E, Eckert A. BDNF in sleep, insomnia, and sleep deprivation. Annals of Medicine. 2016;**48**(1-2):42-51. DOI: 10.3109/07853890.2015.1131327

[41] Shirayama Y, Chen ACH, Nakagawa S, Russell DS, Duman RS. Brain-derived neurotrophic factor produces antidepressant effects in behavioral models of depression. Journal of Neuroscience. 2002;**22**(8):3251-3261. DOI: 10.1523/JNEUROSCI.22-08-03251.2002

[42] Siuciak JA, Lewis DR, Wiegand SJ, Lindsay RM. Antidepressant-like effect of brain-derived neurotrophic factor (BDNF). Pharmacology Biochemistry and Behavior. 1997;**56**(1):131-137. DOI: 10.1016/S0091-3057(96)00169-4

[43] Chen B, Dowlatshahi D, MacQueen GM, Wang JF, Young LT. Increased hippocampal BDNF immunoreactivity in subjects treated with antidepressant medication. Biological Psychiatry. 2001;**50**(4):260-265. DOI: 10.1016/S0006-3223(01)01083-6

[44] Martinowich K, Manji H, Lu B. New insights into BDNF function in depression and anxiety. Nature Neuroscience. 2007;**10**(9):1089-1093. DOI: 10.1038/nn1971

[45] Green MJ, Matheson SL, Shepherd A, Weickert CS, Carr VJ. Brain-derived neurotrophic factor levels in schizophrenia: A systematic review with meta-analysis. Molecular Psychiatry. 2011;**16**(9):960-972. DOI: 10.1038/mp.2010.88

[46] Ströhle A, Stoy M, Graetz B, Scheel M, Wittmann A, Gallinat J, et al. Acute exercise ameliorates reduced brain-derived neurotrophic factor in patients with panic disorder. Psychoneuroendocrinology. 2010;**35**(3):364-368. DOI: 10.1016/j.psyneuen.2009.07.013

[47] Sousa RALD, Improta-Caria AC, Souza BSDF. Exercise–linked irisin: Consequences on mental and cardiovascular health in type 2 diabetes. International Journal of Molecular Sciences. 2021;**22**(4):2199. DOI: 10.3390/ijms22042199

[48] Kurdi FN, Flora R. Physical exercise increased brain-derived neurotrophic factor in elderly population with depression. Open access Macedonian Journal of Medical Sciences. 2019;**7**(13):2057. DOI: 10.3889%2Foamjms.2019.574

[49] Kimhy D, Vakhrusheva J, Bartels MN, Armstrong HF, Ballon JS, Khan S, et al. The impact of aerobic exercise on brain-derived neurotrophic factor and neurocognition in individuals with schizophrenia: A single-blind, randomized clinical trial. Schizophrenia Bulletin. 2015;**41**(4):859-868. DOI: 10.1093/schbul/sbv022

[50] Laske C, Banschbach S, Stransky E, Bosch S, Straten G, Machann J, et al. Exercise-induced normalization of

decreased BDNF serum concentration in elderly women with remitted major depression. International Journal of Neuropsychopharmacology. 2010;**13**(5):595-602. DOI: 10.1017/S1461145709991234

[51] Kerling A, Kück M, Tegtbur U, Grams L, Weber-Spickschen S, Hanke A, et al. Exercise increases serum brain-derived neurotrophic factor in patients with major depressive disorder. Journal of Affective Disorders. 2017;**215**:152-155. DOI: 10.1016/j.jad.2017.03.034

[52] Yeh SH, Lin LW, Chuang YK, Liu CL, Tsai LJ, Tsuei FS, et al. Effects of music aerobic exercise on depression and brain-derived neurotrophic factor levels in community dwelling women. BioMed Research International. 2015;**2015**:135893. DOI: 10.1155/2015/135893. Available from: https://downloads.hindawi.com/journals/bmri/2015/135893.pdf

[53] Hartmann TE, Robertson CV, Miller TD, Hunter JR, Skein M. Associations between exercise, inflammation and symptom severity in those with mental health disorders. Cytokine. 2021;**146**:155648. DOI: 10.1016/j.cyto.2021.155648

[54] Pereira DS, de Queiroz BZ, Miranda AS, Rocha NP, Felício DC, Mateo EC, et al. Effects of physical exercise on plasma levels of brain-derived neurotrophic factor and depressive symptoms in elderly women—A randomized clinical trial. Archives of Physical Medicine and Rehabilitation. 2013;**94**(8):1443-1450. DOI: 10.1016/j.apmr.2013.03.029

[55] Anderson-Hanley C, Barcelos NM, Zimmerman EA, Gillen RW, Dunnam M, Cohen BD, et al. The aerobic and cognitive exercise study (ACES) for community-dwelling older adults with or at-risk for mild cognitive impairment (MCI): Neuropsychological, neurobiological and neuroimaging outcomes of a randomized clinical trial. Frontiers in Aging Neuroscience. 2018;**10**:76. DOI: 10.3389/fnagi.2018.00076

[56] Birinci YZ, Korkmaz NH, Ozturk IE. Can Exergames use as an educational tool in physical education for cognitive, social and affective domains. International Journal of Scientific and Technological Research, Special Issue of Educational Sciences. 2020;**6**(6):151-166. DOI: 10.7176/JSTR/6-06-11

[57] Byun JE, Kang EB. The effects of senior brain health exercise program on basic physical fitness, cognitive function and BDNF of elderly women-a feasibility study. Journal of Exercise Nutrition & Biochemistry. 2016;**20**(2):8. DOI: 10.20463%2Fjenb.2016.06.20.2.2

[58] Kim HJ, Song BK, So B, Lee O, Song W, Kim Y. Increase of circulating BDNF levels and its relation to improvement of physical fitness following 12 weeks of combined exercise in chronic patients with schizophrenia: A pilot study. Psychiatry Research. 2014;**220**(3):792-796. DOI: 10.1016/j.psychres.2014.09.020

[59] McGurk SR, Otto MW, Fulford D, Cutler Z, Mulcahy LP, Talluri SS, et al. A randomized controlled trial of exercise on augmenting the effects of cognitive remediation in persons with severe mental illness. Journal of Psychiatric Research. 2021;**139**:38-46. DOI: 10.1016/j.jpsychires.2021.04.033

[60] Gourgouvelis J, Yielder P, Clarke ST, Behbahani H, Murphy BA. Exercise leads to better clinical outcomes in those receiving medication plus cognitive behavioral therapy for major depressive disorder. Frontiers in

Psychiatry. 2018;**9**:37. DOI: 10.3389/fpsyt.2018.00037

[61] Szuhany KL, Otto MW. Assessing BDNF as a mediator of the effects of exercise on depression. Journal of Psychiatric Research. 2020;**123**:114-118. DOI: 10.1016/j.jpsychires.2020.02.003

[62] Ikai S, Suzuki T, Uchida H, Saruta J, Tsukinoki K, Fujii Y, et al. Effects of weekly one-hour hatha yoga therapy on resilience and stress levels in patients with schizophrenia-spectrum disorders: An eight-week randomized controlled trial. The Journal of Alternative and Complementary Medicine. 2014;**20**(11):823-830. DOI: 10.1089/acm.2014.0205

[63] Szuhany KL, Bugatti M, Otto MW. A meta-analytic review of the effects of exercise on brain-derived neurotrophic factor. Journal of Psychiatric Research. 2015;**60**:56-64. DOI: 10.1016/j.jpsychires.2014.10.003

[64] Marquez CMS, Vanaudenaerde B, Troosters T, Wenderoth N. High-intensity interval training evokes larger serum BDNF levels compared with intense continuous exercise. Journal of Applied Physiology. 2015;**119**:1363-1373. DOI: 10.1152/japplphysiol.00126.2015

[65] Rentería I, García-Suárez PC, Martínez-Corona DO, Moncada-Jiménez J, Plaisance EP, JiméNez-Maldonado A. Short-term high-intensity interval training increases systemic brain-derived neurotrophic factor (BDNF) in healthy women. European Journal of Sport Science. 2020;**20**(4):516-524. DOI: 10.1080/17461391.2019.1650120

[66] Lommatzsch M, Zingler D, Schuhbaeck K, Schloetcke K, Zingler C, Schuff-Werner P, et al. The impact of age, weight and gender on BDNF levels in human platelets and plasma. Neurobiology of Aging. 2005;**26**(1):115-123. DOI: 10.1016/j.neurobiolaging.2004.03.002

[67] Farshbaf M, Alviña K. Multiple roles in neuroprotection for the exercise derived myokine irisin. Frontiers in Aging Neuroscience. 2021;**13**:649929. DOI: 10.3389/fnagi.2021.649929

[68] Bostrom P, Wu J, Jedrychowski MP, Korde A, Ye L, Lo JC, et al. A PGC1-alpha-dependent myokine that drives brown-fat-like development of white fat and thermogenesis. Nature. 2012;**481**:463-468. DOI: 10.1038/nature10777

[69] Aydin S. Three new players in energy regulation: Preptin, adropin and irisin. Peptides. 2014;**56**:94-110. DOI: 10.1016/j.peptides.2014.03.021

[70] Teufel A, Malik N, Mukhopadhyay M, Westphal H. Frcp1 and Frcp2, two novel fibronectin type III repeat containing genes. Gene. 2002;**297**(1-2):79-83. DOI: 10.1016/S0378-1119(02)00828-4

[71] Dun SL, Lyu RM, Chen YH, Chang JK, Luo JJ, Dun NJ. Irisin-immunoreactivity in neural and non-neural cells of the rodent. Neuroscience. 2013;**240**:155-162. DOI: 10.1016/j.neuroscience.2013.02.050

[72] Piya MK, Harte AL, Sivakumar K, Tripathi G, Voyias PD, James S, et al. The identification of irisin in human cerebrospinal fluid: Influence of adiposity, metabolic markers, and gestational diabetes. American Journal of Physiology-Endocrinology and Metabolism. 2014;**306**(5):E512-E518. DOI: 10.1152/ajpendo.00308.2013

[73] Tsuchiya Y, Ando D, Takamatsu K, Goto K. Resistance exercise induces a

greater irisin response than endurance exercise. Metabolism. 2015;**64**(9):1042-1050. DOI: 10.1016/j.metabol.2015.05.010

[74] Kraemer RR, Shockett P, Webb ND, Shah U, Castracane VD. A transient elevated irisin blood concentration in response to prolonged, moderate aerobic exercise in young men and women. Hormone and Metabolic Research. 2014;**46**(02):150-154. DOI: 10.1055/s-0033-1355381

[75] Löffler D, Müller U, Scheuermann K, Friebe D, Gesing J, Bielitz J, et al. Serum irisin levels are regulated by acute strenuous exercise. The Journal of Clinical Endocrinology & Metabolism. 2015;**100**(4):1289-1299. DOI: 10.1210/jc.2014-2932

[76] Jedrychowski MP, Wrann CD, Paulo JA, Gerber KK, Szpyt J, Robinson MM, et al. Detection and quantitation of circulating human irisin by tandem mass spectrometry. Cell Metabolism. 2015;**22**(4):734-740. DOI: 10.1016/j.cmet.2015.08.001

[77] Wrann CD, White JP, Salogiannnis J, Laznik-Bogoslavski D, Wu J, Ma D, et al. Exercise induces hippocampal BDNF through a PGC-1α/FNDC5 pathway. Cell Metabolism. 2013;**18**(5):649-659. DOI: 10.1016/j.cmet.2013.09. 008

[78] Forouzanfar M, Rabiee F, Ghaedi K, Beheshti S, Tanhaei S, Shoaraye Nejati A, et al. Fndc5 overexpression facilitated neural differentiation of mouse embryonic stem cells. Cell Biology International. 2015;**39**(5):629-637. DOI: 10.1002/cbin.10427

[79] Lourenco MV, Frozza RL, de Freitas GB, Zhang H, Kincheski GC, Ribeiro FC, et al. Exercise-linked FNDC5/irisin rescues synaptic plasticity and memory defects in Alzheimer's models. Nature Medicine. 2019;**25**(1):165-175. DOI: 10.1038/s41591-018-0275-4

[80] Cotman CW, Berchtold NC, Christie LA. Exercise builds brain health: Key roles of growth factor cascades and inflammation. Trends in Neurosciences. 2007;**30**(9):464-472. DOI: 10.1016/j.tins.2007.06.011

[81] Mattson MP. Energy intake and exercise as determinants of brain health and vulnerability to injury and disease. Cell Metabolism. 2012;**16**(6):706-722. DOI: 10.1016/j.cmet.2012.08.012

[82] Zheng B, Liao Z, Locascio JJ, Lesniak KA, Roderick SS, Watt ML. & global PD gene expression (GPEX) consortium. Pgc-1 α, a potential therapeutic target for early intervention in parkinson's disease. Science Translational Medicine. 2010;**2**(52):52ra73-52ra73. DOI: 10.1126/scitranslmed.3001059

[83] Yu Q, Li G, Ding Q, Tao L, Li J, Sun L, et al. Irisin protects brain against ischemia/reperfusion injury through suppressing TLR4/MyD88 pathway. Cerebrovascular Diseases. 2020;**49**(4):346-354. DOI: 10.1159/000505961

[84] Leustean L, Preda C, Teodoriu L, Mihalache L, Arhire L, Ungureanu MC. Role of Irisin in endocrine and metabolic disorders—Possible new therapeutic agent? Applied Sciences. 2021;**11**(12):5579. DOI: 10.3390/app11125579

[85] Wang S, Pan J. Irisin ameliorates depressive-like behaviors in rats by regulating energy metabolism. Biochemical and Biophysical Research Communications. 2016;**474**(1):22-28. DOI: 10.1016/j.bbrc.2016.04.047

[86] Wrann CD. FNDC5/Irisin–their role in the nervous system and as a mediator

for beneficial effects of exercise on the brain. Brain Plasticity. 2015;**1**(1):55-61. DOI: 10.3233/BPL-150019

[87] Siteneski A, Cunha MP, Lieberknecht V, Pazini FL, Gruhn K, Brocardo PS, et al. Central irisin administration affords antidepressant-like effect and modulates neuroplasticity-related genes in the hippocampus and prefrontal cortex of mice. Progress in Neuro-Psychopharmacology and Biological Psychiatry. 2018;**84**:294-303. DOI: 10.1016/j.pnpbp.2018.03.004

[88] Tu WJ, Qiu HC, Liu Q, Li X, Zhao JZ, Zeng X. Decreased level of irisin, a skeletal muscle cell-derived myokine, is associated with post-stroke depression in the ischemic stroke population. Journal of Neuroinflammation. 2018;**15**(1):1-10. DOI: 10.1186/s12974-018-1177-6

[89] Szilasi ME, Pak K, Kardos L, Varga VE, Seres I, Mikaczo A, et al. The alteration of Irisin—Brain-derived neurotrophic factor Axis parallels severity of distress disorder in bronchial asthma patients. Frontiers in Neuroscience. 2017;**11**:653. DOI: 10.3389/fnins.2017.00653

[90] Papp C, Pak K, Erdei T, Juhasz B, Seres I, Szentpeteri A, et al. Alteration of the irisin–brain-derived neurotrophic factor axis contributes to disturbance of mood in COPD patients. International Journal of Chronic Obstructive Pulmonary Disease. 2017;**12**:2023. DOI: 10.2147%2FCOPD.S135701

[91] Zsuga J, Tajti G, Papp C, Juhasz B, Gesztelyi R. FNDC5/irisin, a molecular target for boosting reward-related learning and motivation. Medical Hypotheses. 2016;**90**:23-28. DOI: 10.1016/j.mehy.2016.02.020

[92] Han W, Zhang C, Wang H, Yang M, Guo Y, Li G, et al. Alterations of irisin, adropin, preptin and BDNF concentrations in coronary heart disease patients comorbid with depression. Annals of Translational Medicine. 2019 Jul;7(14):298. DOI: 10.21037/atm.2019.05.77

[93] Jo D, Song J. Irisin acts via the PGC-1α and BDNF pathway to improve depression-like behavior. Clinical Nutrition Research. 2021;**10**(4):292. DOI: 10.7762%2Fcnr.2021.10.4.292

[94] Hofmann T, Elbelt U, Ahnis A, Obbarius A, Rose M, Klapp BF, et al. The exercise-induced myokine irisin does not show an association with depressiveness, anxiety and perceived stress in obese women. Journal of Physiology and Pharmacology: An Official Journal of the Polish Physiological Society. 2016;**67**(2):195-203 PMID: 27226179

[95] Dyer AH, Vahdatpour C, Sanfeliu A, Tropea D. The role of insulin-like growth factor 1 (IGF-1) in brain development, maturation and neuroplasticity. Neuroscience. 2016;**325**:89-99. DOI: 10.1016/j.neuroscience.2016.03.056

[96] Deak F, Sonntag WE. Aging, synaptic dysfunction, and insulin-like growth factor (IGF)-1. Journals of Gerontology Series A: Biomedical Sciences and Medical Sciences. 2012;**67**(6):611-625. DOI: 10.1093/gerona/gls118

[97] Gubbi S, Quipildor GF, Barzilai N, Huffman DM, Milman S. 40 YEARS of IGF1: IGF1: The Jekyll and Hyde of the aging brain. Journal of Molecular Endocrinology. 2018;**61**(1):T171-T185. DOI: 10.1530/JME-18-0093

[98] Åberg ND, Brywe KG, Isgaard J. Aspects of growth hormone and

insulin-like growth factor-I related to neuroprotection, regeneration, and functional plasticity in the adult brain. TheScientificWorldJOURNAL. 2006;**6**:53-80. DOI: 10.1100/tsw.2006.22

[99] Herold F, Törpel A, Schega L, Müller NG. Functional and/or structural brain changes in response to resistance exercises and resistance training lead to cognitive improvements–a systematic review. European Review of Aging and Physical Activity. 2019;**16**(1):1-33. DOI: 10.1186/s11556-019-0217-2

[100] Calvo D, Gunstad J, Miller LA, Glickman E, Spitznagel MB. Higher serum insulin-like growth factor-1 is associated with better cognitive performance in persons with mild cognitive impairment. Psychogeriatrics. 2013;**13**(3):170-174. DOI: 10.1111/psyg.12023

[101] Duron E, Funalot B, Brunel N, Coste J, Quinquis L, Viollet C, et al. Insulin-like growth factor-I and insulin-like growth factor binding protein-3 in Alzheimer's disease. The Journal of Clinical Endocrinology & Metabolism. 2012;**97**(12):4673-4681. DOI: 10.1210/jc.2012-2063

[102] Stein AM, da Silva TMV, de Melo Coelho FG, Rueda AV, Camarini R, Galduróz RFS. Acute exercise increases circulating IGF-1 in Alzheimer's disease patients, but not in older adults without dementia. Behavioural Brain Research. 2021;**396**:112903. DOI: 10.1016/j.bbr.2020.112903

[103] de Alcantara Borba D, da Silva Alves E, Rosa JPP, Facundo LA, Costa CMA, Silva AC, et al. Can IGF-1 serum levels really be changed by acute physical exercise? A systematic review and meta-analysis. Journal of Physical Activity and Health. 2020;**17**(5):575-584. DOI: 10.1123/jpah.2019-0453

[104] Cassilhas RC, Antunes HKM, Tufik S, De Mello MT. Mood, anxiety, and serum IGF-1 in elderly men given 24 weeks of high resistance exercise. Perceptual and Motor Skills. 2010;**110**(1):265-276. DOI: 10.2466%2Fpms.110.1.265-276

[105] Yoon JR, Ha GC, Kang SJ, Ko KJ. Effects of 12-week resistance exercise and interval training on the skeletal muscle area, physical fitness, and mental health in old women. Journal of Exercise Rehabilitation. 2019;**15**(6):839. DOI: 10.12965%2Fjer.1938644.322

[106] Tsai CL, Ukropec J, Ukropcová B, Pai MC. An acute bout of aerobic or strength exercise specifically modifies circulating exerkine levels and neurocognitive functions in elderly individuals with mild cognitive impairment. NeuroImage: Clinical. 2018;**17**:272-284. DOI: 10.1016/j.nicl.2017.10.028

[107] Ding Q, Vaynman S, Akhavan M, Ying Z, Gomez-Pinilla F. Insulin-like growth factor I interfaces with brain-derived neurotrophic factor-mediated synaptic plasticity to modulate aspects of exercise-induced cognitive function. Neuroscience. 2006;**140**(3):823-833. DOI: 10.1016/j.neuroscience.2006.02.084

[108] Carro E, Nuñez A, Busiguina S, Torres-Aleman I. Circulating insulin-like growth factor I mediates effects of exercise on the brain. Journal of Neuroscience. 2000;**20**(8):2926-2933. DOI: 10.1523/JNEUROSCI.20-08-02926.2000

[109] Agid Y, Buzsáki G, Diamond DM, Frackowiak R, Giedd J, Girault JA, et al. How can drug discovery for psychiatric disorders be improved? Nature Reviews Drug Discovery. 2007;**6**(3):189-201. DOI: 10.1038/nrd2217

[110] De Sousa RAL, Improta-Caria AC, Aras-Júnior R, de Oliveira EM, Soci ÚPR, Cassilhas RC. Physical exercise effects on the brain during COVID-19 pandemic: Links between mental and cardiovascular health. Neurological Sciences. 2021;**42**(4):1325-1334. DOI: 10.1007/s10072-021-05082-9

[111] Stimpson NJ, Davison G, Javadi AH. Joggin'the noggin: Towards a physiological understanding of exercise-induced cognitive benefits. Neuroscience & Biobehavioral Reviews. 2018;**88**:177-186. DOI: 10.1016/j.neubiorev.2018.03.018

[112] Duric V, Duman RS. (2013). Depression and treatment response: Dynamic interplay of signaling pathways and altered neural processes. Cellular and Molecular Life Sciences. 2013;**70**(1):39-53. DOI: 10.1007/s00018-012-1020-7

[113] Clark-Raymond A, Meresh E, Hoppensteadt D, Fareed J, Sinacore J, Halaris A. Vascular endothelial growth factor: A potential diagnostic biomarker for major depression. Journal of Psychiatric Research. 2014;**59**:22-27. DOI: 10.1016/j.jpsychires.2014.08.005

[114] Kuga GK, Botezelli JD, Gaspar RC, Gomes RJ, Pauli JR, Leme JACDA. Hippocampal insulin signaling and neuroprotection mediated by physical exercise in Alzheimer´ s disease. Motriz: Revista de Educação Física. 2017;**23**:e101608. DOI: 10.1590/S1980-6574201700SI0008. Available from: https://www.scielo.br/j/motriz/a/MKLTSzctmbPK9b9RSQsGNDd/?format=pdf&lang=en

[115] Elemery M, Lazary J, Kiss S, Dome P, Pogany L, Faludi G. Change of circulating vascular endothelial growth factor (VEGF) level and reduction of anhedonia is associated in patients with major depressive disorder treated with rTMS. Frontiers in Psychiatry. 2022;**13**:1021. DOI: 10.3389/fpsyt.2022.806731

[116] Halmai Z, Dome P, Dobos J, Gonda X, Szekely A, Sasvari-Szekely M, et al. Peripheral vascular endothelial growth factor level is associated with antidepressant treatment response: Results of a preliminary study. Journal of Affective Disorders. 2013;**144**(3):269-273. DOI: 10.1016/j.jad.2012.09.006

[117] Matsuno H, Tsuchimine S, O'Hashi K, Sakai K, Hattori K, Hidese S, et al. Association between vascular endothelial growth factor-mediated blood–brain barrier dysfunction and stress-induced depression. Molecular Psychiatry. 2022:1-11. DOI: 10.1038/s41380-022-01618-3. Available from: https://www.nature.com/articles/s41380-022-01618-3

[118] Hadidi N, Treat-Jacobson DJ, Lindquist R. Poststroke depression and functional outcome: A critical review of literature. Heart & Lung. 2009;**38**(2):151-162. DOI: 10.1016/j.hrtlng.2008.05.002

[119] Udo H, Hamasu K, Furuse M, Sugiyama H. VEGF-induced antidepressant effects involve modulation of norepinephrine and serotonin systems. Behavioural Brain Research. 2014;**275**:107-113. DOI: 10.1016/j.bbr.2014.09.005

[120] Morland C, Andersson KA, Haugen ØP, Hadzic A, Kleppa L, Gille A, et al. Exercise induces cerebral VEGF and angiogenesis via the lactate receptor HCAR1. Nature Communications. 2017;**8**(1):1-9. DOI: 10.1038/ncomms15557

[121] Schobersberger W, Hobisch-Hagen P, Fries D, Wiedermann F, Rieder-Scharinger J, Villiger B, et al.

Increase in immune activation, vascular endothelial growth factor and erythropoietin after an ultramarathon run at moderate altitude. Immunobiology. 2000;**201**(5):611-620. DOI: 10.1016/S0171-2985(00)80078-9

[122] Ma C, Lin M, Gao J, Xu S, Huang L, Zhu J, et al. The impact of physical activity on blood inflammatory cytokines and neuroprotective factors in individuals with mild cognitive impairment: A systematic review and meta-analysis of randomized-controlled trials. Aging Clinical and Experimental Research. 2022;**34**:1-14. DOI: 10.1007/s40520-021-02069-6

[123] Krogh J, Rostrup E, Thomsen C, Elfving B, Videbech P, Nordentoft M. The effect of exercise on hippocampal volume and neurotrophines in patients with major depression–a randomized clinical trial. Journal of Affective Disorders. 2014;**165**:24-30. DOI: 10.1016/j.jad.2014.04.041

[124] Tsai CL, Pai MC, Ukropec J, Ukropcová B. Distinctive effects of aerobic and resistance exercise modes on neurocognitive and biochemical changes in individuals with mild cognitive impairment. Current Alzheimer Research. 2019;**16**(4):316-332. DOI: 10.2174/1567205016666190228125429

[125] Du X, Chen W, Zhan N, Bian X, Yu W. The effects of low-intensity resistance training with or without blood flow restriction on serum BDNF, VEGF and perception in patients with post-stroke depression. Neuroendocrinology Letters. 2021;**42**(4):229-235

[126] Kim S, Choi JY, Moon S, Park DH, Kwak HB, Kang JH. Roles of myokines in exercise-induced improvement of neuropsychiatric function. Pflügers Archiv-European Journal of Physiology. 2019;**471**(3):491-505. DOI: 10.1007/s00424-019-02253-8

[127] Phillips C, Fahimi A. Immune and neuroprotective effects of physical activity on the brain in depression. Frontiers in Neuroscience. 2018;**12**:498. DOI: 10.3389/fnins.2018.00498

[128] Voelcker-Rehage C, Niemann C. Structural and functional brain changes related to different types of physical activity across the life span. Neuroscience Biobehavioral. Reviews. 2013;**37**:2268-2295. DOI: 10.1016/j.neubiorev.2013.01.028

[129] Perlis RH. Exercising heart and head in managing coronavirus disease 2019 in Wuhan. JAMA Network Open. 2020;**3**(3):e204006-e204006. DOI: 10.1001/jamanetworkopen.2020.4006

[130] Birinci YZ, Korkmaz NH, Deniz M, Pancar S, Çetinoglu G, Topçu H. The effects of Exergames on the attitudes of secondary school female students towards physical education. Journal of Educational Issues. 2021;**7**(3):291-300. DOI: 10.5296/jei.v7i3.19187

Chapter 4

# Exploring the Effectiveness of Mental Health First Aid Program for Young People in South Africa

*Chinwe Christopher Obuaku-Igwe*


## Abstract

This study explored the effectiveness of a mental health first-aid program on improving young people's attitudes, knowledge and mental health-related behavior, using qualitative methods. An assessment of the pilot project that was conducted among social science students between age 18 and 34 years revealed a reduction in stigma, increased openness about mental health challenges and increase in utilization of professional services among participants (n-548) of the MHFA program, following the 13-week program. The study found that MHFA intervention projects were considerably more effective in changing attitudes towards mental illness when blended with indigenous concepts, values, language, as well as priorities for various cultures and settings. Based on analysis of course content and focused group discussions, the study concludes that four factors contributed to the overwhelming satisfaction experienced by participants: (1) the utilization of peer tutors in administering the training, (2) the inclusion of mental models and centering participants' agency in creating and administering training content, (3) the availability of peer mentors and a mobile application which makes referral (social prescribing) and access to professional intervention easy, and (4) the inclusion of friends and family as accountability partners.


**Keywords:** mental health first aid, South Africa, cultural competence, health education, mental illness

## 1. Introduction

This paper provides an overview of the investigation of the effectiveness of a Mental Health First Aid program hereafter known as MHFA, among young people between the age of 18 and 30 years in South Africa. There is growing evidence of the efficiency of mental health first aid in the Global North, specifically, in the United States of America [1] and the United Kingdom [2]. However, the implementation of MHFA programs in these contexts were embedded within broader national health intervention projects. In this sense, MHFA programs were utilized and implemented within broader social prescribing [3] or community referral systems where trained health professionals referred individuals to various categories of nonclinical services. There is growing evidence that MHFA holds potential for de-stigmatization and improved access to professional services within rural [4] or low-resource settings, even when such programs are designed outside national clinical settings.

It is known that the earlier an individual receives support or intervention, the higher their chances of recovery from a mental illness. Within this context, further studies are required to investigate how effective nonprofit organization (NPO)- or community-led MHFA programs have been in improving attitudes, knowledge, and general mental health-related behavior among young people. Mental Health First Aid (MHFA) is an adaptation of physical first-aid training [5], for emotional or psychological health emergencies. It emerged out of the need to provide immediate support for individuals experiencing mental health crises. Drawing on this, researchers [6] explain that MHFA involves a six-step process of approaching an individual experiencing a mental health crisis: assessing and assisting with the crisis; listening and communicating with them without prejudice or; providing support and information; encouraging the individual to get appropriate professional help; and encouraging other forms of support.

MHFA involves a process of increasing participant's knowledge of mental wellbeing in order to increase supportive attitude while reducing their negative behavior toward individuals experiencing mental health challenges [7]. Mental health literacy is a broad term that involves reducing negative behaviors and increasing support for people with mental illness. Therefore, as an adaptation of the physical first-aid training which emerged out of the interlinked processes of providing a first point of contact to help individuals with mental health challenges, MHFA is a kind of support offered to an individual experiencing a mental health crisis until the appropriate professional help is received or until the crisis is resolved [8]. This could be individuals who have experienced a major traumatic event or are suicidal.

Mental Health First Aid International [9] notes that this physiological emergency support began in 2000, in Australia, through the collaborative efforts of a researcher and a part-time volunteer who had experienced mental health issues. Jorm and Kitchener [10] note that by 2011, there were over 850 instructors in Australia who had trained over 170,000 adults. As of July 2022, MHFA is being delivered in 24 countries by over 60,000 accredited instructors and over 5 million people who have received training. Within this framework, MHFA targets mostly individuals in professions or environments with high probability of interacting with people experiencing mental health emergencies such as parents, youth group leaders, police officers, coaches, social workers, camp counselors, teachers, family caregivers, and other individuals who work with the youth among others.

Understanding the effectiveness of MHFA involves a process of contextualizing it within and across specific political, cultural, and socioeconomic contexts [11]. However, not much is known about MHFA implementation mechanisms in the Global South. Even though MHFA has been adapted to various disasters and populations in different countries and regions, detailed knowledge of the basic principles surrounding its adaptations by various stakeholders in South Africa remains under-researched and inadequately known. The processes of MHFA implementation such as the duration of implementation, content, for whom it was intended, identity of tutors implementing it, circumstances under which MHFA was administered, where they administered it, and how and at what cost MHFA was administered have not been a subject of research in South Africa. Yet, there exists a substantial body of contextual work in psychology, social work, nursing, pharmacy, and the biomedical sciences on psychological first aid [12–14]. These studies have been concerned with identifying the characteristics, participants of MHFA programs, and the contexts of their implementation.

The research focus differs significantly reflecting the heterogeneity of interests, aims, viewpoints, and approach of researchers. For example, a scoping review which was conducted in 2020 [14] focused on mapping MHFA programs to contextualize its implementation mechanisms across various contexts, NG et al. [12] in their systematic review, concentrated on youth and teen MHFA, exploring the body of work that describes its delivery and assessment among university students as well as discipline and participants' level of study. Another systematic review [13] which focused on summarizing the current evidence for youth and teen MHFA in order to provide direction for future training and research concluded that there was a need for more empirical research in non-Western countries, high-risk populations, and different professional settings. They noted that future interventions could also consider different modes of learning, longer-term follow-up, and the measurement of outcomes that evaluate the quality of helping behavior. These existing bodies of literature that describe the assessment and delivery of MHFA training among college students revealed that while MHFA was not compulsory for most students in healthcare professions, of those enrolled in the program within the United States, Australia, and United Kingdom, majority were pharmacy, healthcare, and social work majors.

Furthermore, disciplines who implemented MHFA training integrated the adult version into their curriculum and made it mandatory for all students across all years of their program, focusing mostly on mental health literacy, confidence, stigma, knowledge, intentions, and application of skills. In addition, while most of these programs assessed participants based on their knowledge of skills related to mental health literacy, only a few focused on self-reported health measurements and direct observation of behaviors. MHFA can be thought of as a first-aid box for the mind, used to recognize symptoms of physiological distress and to provide initial support and treatment. Hart, Jorm, Paxton, and Cvetkovski [15] note that MHFA needs to be situated beyond healthcare and "care" spaces in order to understand its positive impact on participants.

Given the current trend for MHFA certification requirements for adult professionals within care roles and occupation in the Global North, it is not surprising that disciplines within biomedical sciences and public health now integrate MHFA as a compulsory aspect of their programs across all levels. However, the context of the implementation of the tertiary MHFA program among students within the social sciences and its impact on both instructors and students in the Global South is unclear. For example, the full scope and context of MHFA adaptation in South Africa is unclear. In addition, it is not clear whether MHFA programs adapted by nonprofit organizations (NPOs) for social science majors within low-income settings lead to mental health literacy, improved support, de-stigmatization, and access to professional services [16]. Although, mental health issues have significant impact on countries and individual's financial wellbeing, productivity, and life expectancy, with an estimated economic cost of over USD$ 16.1 trillion from the global economy between 2010 and 2030 [17].

A MHFA training impact assessment study [18] conducted among 166 adult participants who enrolled in classes organized by a community health center in rural Kansas in the United States reported that even though the response rate was low (36%) for the online feedback survey, there was evidence of changed behaviors, attitudes, and improved mental health literacy. However, as with most impact assessments, there were suggestions for additional research to better understand change processes that occur as a result of MHFA across multicultural and diverse settings within and outside the United States. Noltemeyer et al. [19] assessed the impact of a national rollout of Youth Mental Health First Aid (YMHFA) training among adults in Ohio who were trained as first responders to youth in crisis. The pilot study utilized data gathered from over 2180 predominantly White women within the education sector. They found significant improvements in self-confidence, openness to individuals with mental health conditions, willingness to help, and awareness of mental wellbeing resources and support, 3 months after training.

The MHFAI [20] notes that its global presence is currently limited to 26 countries, mostly within the Global North, with the exception of India and Bangladesh. While international uptake for MHFA within the Global South and Africa in particular appears developmental, evaluations of its effectiveness and benefits of current programs among individuals and communities within these contexts are scarce. In fact, proponents of MHFA training suggest the need for further partnership with research (and researchers) as its international uptake and perceptions of its effectiveness depend largely on access to evidence-based evaluative publication. When considered as a body of work, evidence-based evaluative publications on MHFA particularly, within the Global South is scarce and inconclusive. In addition, there is limited empirical work on the effectiveness of MHFA in Africa and its cultural appropriateness.

A Delphi expert consensus study which reviewed guidelines for providing mental health first aid to suicidal individuals in India, against the backdrop of growing suicide, noted that while their target population were mental health professionals, the program could be adapted outside its intended context, for individuals who work in welfare and health settings as well as ethnic minorities. The reviewers [21] suggested that it was imperative to evaluate the impact of such guidelines on the first aider's helping behavior and on the recipients of the first aid. The evaluation would assist researchers in developing an evidence base for mental health first aid and suicide prevention initiatives. Another Delphi expert consensus study which reviewed a cultural adaptation of the mental health first-aid guidelines for assisting people at risk of suicide in Brazil supported the importance of adapting the guidelines to various cultures. They found that the incorporation of aspects of Brazilian culture such as family and friends and self-care for first-aid providers helped in improving health outcomes.

However, a mixed-methods study [22] of an advocacy program for mental healthcare users in South Africa which evaluated the implementation of a national advocacy program for mental healthcare users, conducted by the South African National Department of Health and the South African Federation for Mental Health, reported that although the programs helped with mental health literacy there was inadequate support from NGOs or the Department of Health (DoH), which impeded sustainability of mental health advocacy efforts. They noted scarcity of professional mental health services in primary care clinics, with acute care limited to provincial tertiary hospitals, where the majority of resources are allocated. The study concluded that limited resource allocation and prioritization of mental disorders within the South African public health system created inequities in access to treatment which has now resulted in human suffering, disability, and economic losses [23].

Globally, young people and women have the highest rate of global emotional disorder [24]. One in six people between 17 to 19 years have a mental disorder with 1 in 16 experiencing more than one mental disorder in 2017. Fifty percent of all lifetime mental illness begins by the age of 14 years and 75% by the age of 24 years [25]. In South Africa, the statistics are similar. A report from the South African Federation for Mental Health (SAFMH) [26] on the state of mental health in the country indicated that in 2o18, 18% of learners in the country (between ages 15 to 19 years) reported having suicide ideation, 18% had attempted suicide, 25% reported experiencing

*DOI: http://dx.doi.org/10.5772/intechopen.108303*

feelings of hopelessness and sadness, and 32% of those who attempted suicide required medical treatment. Yet, the optimal methods of promoting health and the effectiveness of MHFA with young people in South Africa are not clear. However, research and interventions in other areas have shown that more awareness, MHFA, and community participation decrease the stigma and therefore increase the chances of getting help.

The SAFMH and SADAG [27] noted the absence of a national MHFA guide, explaining that even though NGOs, communities, and other nongovernmental agencies were implementing mental health literacy and first-aid interventions within their various communities, the culturally appropriateness of those programs were unclear. They suggested that formulating laws or policies and funding evaluative research efforts that provided specific step-by-step advocacy guidelines on how to mitigate mental health crises or cater specifically for the needs of this demographic would contribute to addressing these health issues in an evidence-based manner. It thus remains to be seen whether MHFA efforts by NGOs in South Africa, in the absence of a national guide, are culturally appropriate and effective among the most vulnerable social groups. In light of growing international uptake of MHFA and the need to understand its full scope and the cultural appropriateness of implementation mechanisms for its tertiary guidelines, among young people, this paper forms part of the broader attempt at investigating the effectiveness of MHFA in South Africa.

It focuses specifically, on MHFA in the Western Cape province of South Africa, to examine the extent and degree to which an NPO (nonprofit organization) has included protective factors in its adaptation of MHFA among social science majors, aged 18 to 34 years in the Western Cape province of South Africa. The paper delimits its focus to self-reported measurements of the impact of MHFA training on both peer trainers and trainees. Within this context, the aim of the current study is twofold: to describe the scope and characteristics of an NPO-led MHFA program in the Western Cape province of South Africa and secondly, to assess the cultural appropriateness and effectiveness of adapted guidelines on participants and the extent to which it is useful in mental wellbeing management (using self-reported health measurement).

## 2. Methods

### 2.1 Indima Yethu's pilot project

Despite its growing popularity as a method of improving mental literacy and wellbeing, national uptake of MHFA in South Africa has been slow, as with other mental health related policies in the country. In the absence of a well-coordinated national MHFA strategy, guidelines, and agenda, the responsibility for mental health literacy has fallen on civil societies and communities. These organizations and communities design and pilot adapted MHFA training nationally, based on assumptions that are drawn from international research from the Global North, which leaves gaps in perceptions and understanding of the cultural appropriateness of MHFA training in South Africa. This paper examines the outcome of a culturally adapted version of MHFA in South Africa (which included spirituality and ubuntu values), implemented by a nonprofit organization, Indima Yethu. The current assessment of outcomes form part of a wider effort at building an evidence base of the utilization of YMHFA in South Africa, through a post-training feedback interview of MHFA participants in Cape Town.

Since 2018, Indima Yethu has been working with children and young people (CYP) in providing participatory health promotion interventions and culturally adapted MHFA training. In view of the complex mental health issues facing the South African youth during and post-lockdown, the NPO developed a 13-week YMHFA program, for over 863 young people aged 18–34 years, across the Western Cape province in South Africa, to enable them serve as first responders to their peers who were in crisis.

The foundation to Indima Yethu's Youth MHFA program was laid for the first time by a needs assessment survey which revealed that a number of factors put students and young people at risk of writing – anxiety, panic attacks, paranoia, and depression. Among these factors are mismatched expectations, poor socioeconomic status, and uneven ratio of psychologists to students at various universities in South Africa.

Based on these, the goal of Indima Yethu's MHFA training program is to create an informal peer mentoring and mental health support group to fill the gaps.

Thus, working from an asset-based theoretical and a participatory health research framework, the MHFA training program provides a space where students and other participants are able to improve their writing skills and manage their mental health and that of their peers who have no access to professional support through shared narrative therapy or mental health first aid. The methods and intervention tools utilized by Indima Yethu are underpinned by research-backed philosophy that writing, journaling, and narrative therapy give coherence and increase mindfulness, while peer support is cathartic and eases anxiety. Thus, Indima Yethu's MHFA trainings were held online and offline (onsite at their Cape Town office) once a week for 2 hours each, over a 13-week period per session. The broader goals were summarized thus:

i. Creativity—to help unlock the student's creativity and let it flow by learning self-expression.

ii. Self-discipline and willpower—To help students solve problems by tracking personal patterns of behavior, being honest with themselves about what they feel per day, why and to become their first critic in a safe environment—their journals.

iii. Improve problem solving abilities—Through journaling, writing personal narratives and peer support, students can take the edge off toxic emotions and gain clarity on future steps they need to take, while looking back on their writing to see progress made—how far they have come, how they handled challenges, and what personal patterns become roadblocks in their personal and professional life.

iv. Stress reduction and improved memory—For students to stop letting their thoughts control them negatively. For them to be goal-oriented and let their goals drive them toward taking little steps that would culminate in success in any aspect of their lives.

v. Self-awareness and mindfulness—For the students to come to terms with the things they can control and those outside their control and through that recognize the sources of their anxiety and dissatisfaction with life.

### 2.2 Research design and procedures

The context for the current research was an NPO, Indima Yethu, located in Cape Town, whose work focuses on youth mentoring, capacity development, health promotion, and advocacy. Working with Indima Yethu, the data for this study were collected from the Indima Yethu Youth Mental Health First Aid program with ethics number HS21/5/65 from the University of the Western Cape. The data were collected from an analysis of records, intensive observation, and focused group interviews administered between October 2021 and June 2022, by a researcher from the University of the Western Cape. The sampling area was the Western Cape province, and sampling was a three-stage process. In the first stage, all trainees who had participated in the Indima Yethu 13-week Youth Mental Health First Aid program were selected based on a convenience sampling (n = 862). In the second stage, individuals who had participated in the program and utilized the referral system via the mental health app (sentinel) or through a mental health first-aid instructor were included. In the final stage, participants were selected from the second sample, including people who had trained, completed, and graduated from the 13-week course before, during, and after the lockdown as well as those who had lived experience of any form of mental illness.

I used broad categories to cover each group discussion as well as specific open-ended and closed-ended questions that focused on mental literacy and other determinants of wellbeing such as security, health, safety, employment, living conditions, housing, economy, leisure, civic activities, and social relationships. The reason for exploring these broad themes was to ensure that significant aspects of the research were covered during group discussions. In line with my grounding in these frameworks, I adopted a collaborative, consultative, and unstructured approach to the group discussions. As noted by Chevalier & Buckles [28], participatory approaches to research have the potential to facilitate solutions and avert conflicts between individuals in a group setting. They note that aside enhancing data reliability and validity, these approaches also increase researcher's ability to identify and highlight assets within communities while helping them find solutions and develop strong partnerships.

Participants were required to respond to survey questions which were emailed by the program organizers. The email contained a cover letter, a link to the survey, and an invitation to participate in the FGDs workshop where the group discussions were held. The weekly workshops were conducted face to face and online. The weekly focused group discussions were facilitated by the author due to her experience in the pilot and cross-cultural study. I took notes during the weekly workshop sessions to document thought patterns and encourage reflexivity. Participants were divided into 4-hour sessions twice a week, over 13 weeks. They were required to participate in at least one session per week. The total number of hours spent facilitating discussions with participants was 104 hours. The categories for the lines of inquiries for the group discussions were generated from an extensive reading of literature and focused on each aspect of the surveys as well. Informed consent was obtained from participants after the aims of the study were explained to them.

### 2.3 Post-MHFA course survey

As earlier indicated, online surveys and focused group workshops were the primary data collection tools. These data collection tools were designed to assess participants' perceptions, behaviors, knowledge, and attitudes toward mental illness, spirituality, level of empathy, coping mechanisms, and other protective factors for mental wellbeing. The assessment survey for participants took 10 minutes to complete on Google doc form and included 20 MCQs and other demographic data-related questions that required short responses. Although the lines of inquiry and survey questions were teased out from a review of MHFA literature and in consultation with instructors at Indima Yethu, in order to establish content validity, they were submitted to participants of the Indima Yethu MHFA course and other MHFA program organizers for feedback. Feedback from participants and experts were particularly important to me as I was working from an evaluative ubuntu, asset-based, participatory and decolonial epistemological and theoretical framework.

The survey items included four broad themes: the first theme covered the demographic profile of participants such as educational background, age, gender, ethnicity/race, socio-economic status, mental health lived experience, coping mechanism, etc.; the second theme assessed changes in participant's knowledge by focusing on their ability to gain and utilize newly acquired mental literacy information upon completion of the MHFA training; the third theme focused on change in attitude and helping behavior toward others; the fourth theme assessed Indima Yethu YMHFA 13-week module-related outcomes which asked questions related to spirituality, confidence, and self-esteem. For questions that fell within themes two and three, participants were required to rate statements using a five-point Likert scales (The response scale for items in categories 2 to 4 were 1 (strongly disagree), 2 (agree), 3 (neutral), 4 (agree), 5 (Strongly agree), and 6 (other).

Each item was meant to indicate the response that best captured the effectiveness of the MHFA program and participants attitudes toward applying the ALGEE action plan:

1. Assess for risk of suicide or harm.

2. Listen non-judgmentally.

3. Give reassurance and information.

4. Encourage appropriate professional help and

5. Encourage self-help and other support strategies

Most of the questions were adapted from existing literature and previous studies on the outcome assessment of MHFA training, and some of the statements participants rated include "I remember ALGEE," "I have utilized and applied ALGEE action plan," "I remember the MHFA course content and can teach my peers," "I have utilized and applied the MHFA course content for myself," "I have utilized and applied the MHFA course content for my family," "I have utilized and applied the MHFA course content in my community," "I have applied the YMHFA training content in my everyday life," "I learned new information about mental disorders in the YMHFA course," "I am now confident in helping an individual experiencing a mental health challenge as a result of the YMHFA course," "My behavior towards mental disorders has changed as a result of the MHFA course," "My attitude towards mentally ill people has changed as a result of the MHFA course," "I am more eager to help my community destigmatize mental illness", etc.

Items that fell within theme four which focused on Indima Yethu's specific resources such as spirituality, self-confidence, de-stigmatization and self-esteem, and participants were required to circle the responses that indicate how the 13-week MHFA course from Indima Yethu impacted their wellbeing, that of their loved ones and their openness to spirituality. The response scale for these items were rated as positive or negative using a 5-point scale: 1 (very favorable), 2 (favorable), 3 (very unfavorable), 4 (unfavorable), and 5 (NA). Furthermore, participants were asked to indicate how often they were in contact with other individuals experiencing mental health crises and to describe how they supported them as well as their level of confidence in their ability to support others. If they indicated that they had helped someone while taking the course or after, they were asked to list the number of times and under what circumstance they made referrals using Indima Yethu's in-house mobile app. Participants used the focused group workshop platforms to unpack all responses provided in the surveys.

### 2.4 Participants

Overall, a total of 548 young people aged 18 to 34 years participated in the study, having completed the YMHFA program through Indima Yethu between December 2019 and June 2022. Of all participants, the general response rate was 98%. Overall, 76.3% of participants were females (n = 418), with a median age of 21.5 years, 87.2% were single, and 57.7% were colored (n = 316) with 38.3% Black Africans (n = 210) and approximately 1.8% (n = 10) Whites. Seventy-nine percent (n = 426) of participants had high school diplomas at the time they underwent the training, and others were mostly social science and humanities undergraduate majors enrolled at various universities in the Western Cape with no prior training in healthcare. Almost all participants had experienced one form of mental illness or had a close family member or friend who had. Approximately 62.2% (n = 341) of participants reported that their annual household income was below R100,000 (equivalent to 6116 US Dollars when controlled for inflation).

### 2.5 Data analysis

Considering the prevalence of quantitative research on MHFA, the current study will prioritize qualitative insights in order to unpack, enrich, and add the much-needed depth to this emerging topic. All focused group discussions were audio-recorded, transcribed, and coded manually. The process of coding and content analysis enabled us to highlight similarities in experiences. It also enabled us to link quantitative data with qualitative insights and patterns that were generated as well as explain them. This process allowed one to generate major patterns, themes, and concepts [29]. Descriptive statistics are used to categorize and summarize demographic data from participants, and content analysis was used to summarize qualitative data emerging from the FGD on the perceived outcomes of the ALGEE action plan, changes in attitudes and knowledge, supportive behavior, mental health literacy, and spirituality. The pilot study (Obuaku-Igwe, 2020) that preceded the current one generated baseline information on protective factors for mental wellbeing among young people in South Africa. It is anticipated that the current study will yield further information on the effectiveness of MHFA as a protective factor in mental wellbeing management among young people in informal settlements in the Western Cape, for further studies of the social welfare and social protection of CYP in South Africa.

See table one below for further details about participants' mental health experiences and coping mechanisms before the MHFA training (**Table 1**).

### 2.6 Results

Content analysis of focused group discussions utilized a bottom-up [30] approach where I tried to identify phrases that were related to broad categories linked to

| Mental illness | n | % |
|---|---|---|
| Anxiety/depression | 365 | 70.6 |
| Bipolar | 99 | 18.1 |
| Eating disorder | 62 | 11.3 |
| Coping mechanism for mental illness prior to enrollment in MHFA at Indima Yethu | | |
| Coping mechanism | n | % |
| Music | 273 | 49.8 |
| Weed | 129 | 23.5 |
| Energy drink | 109 | 19.9 |
| Alcohol | 37 | 6.8 |

**Table 1.**
*Participants lived experience of mental disorder and coping mechanism before MHFA (N = 548).*

changes in behavior due to utilization of new knowledge, helping behavior, and increase in self-confidence. Afterward, I organized all relevant statements into repetitive themes below the broader categories of changes in behavior, helping behavior, and increase in self-confidence.

### *2.6.1 Knowledge retention and utilization*

Questions under the first theme assessed the extent to which participants' attitudes changed due to acquisition and utilization of new knowledge through the YMHFA training program. 75.5% of the participants (n = 414) reported that upon completion of the training that they remembered and have utilized aspects of the ALGEE course content and a few people (24.5%, n = 134) indicated that they did not remember much. Of those who remembered the YMHFA course content, majority (81.6%, n = 447) indicated that they utilized the knowledge gained in recognizing signs of mental health issues and instability in their lives and among friends and family members and 17.9% (n = 98) utilized the knowledge of ALGEE in helping colleagues at work.

Overwhelmingly, participants with lived experiences of anxiety/depression who used weed, energy drink, and alcohol as coping mechanisms reported a decline in their utilization of substances after taking the MHFA training. They had accepted the construction of their illness and stigma attached to it by family regardless of how it made them feel, but the training helped in changing their perception of mental illness. Most notably, those with lived experiences of bipolar disorder journaled more during the 13-week training and viewed music as a good coping mechanism each time they felt overwhelmed. The participants with eating disorders differed greatly from other participants, noting that the module on embodied experiences changed their mental models and helped them in overcoming fears about eating and overall construction of selfhood.

### *2.6.2 Changes in helping attitude due to mental health literacy*

The range of questions within this category assessed various ways in which participants' helping behavior has changed post-training. A good number of participants

75.7% (n = 415) indicated that prior to the training sessions, they did not know about MHFA and only 22.8%(n = 125) said they were familiar with MHFA as a concept. Majority of participants (84.8%, n = 465) indicated that they acquired new knowledge from the training which changed their behavior toward mentally ill people as well as their perceptions of mental disorders. 75.9% (n = 416) indicated that the training they received improved their understanding of the risks associated with untreated mental illness; 16.6% (n = 91) were neutral and only 7.5% (n = 41) said they did not know the risk factors. 87% (n = 477) indicated that upon completing the training, they have become more aware of the prevalence of mental illness among their peers and have experienced individuals with emotional distress whom they supported through referrals and other ALGEE strategies. Of those who provided some form of support for individuals with mental illness, 65.4% (n = 358) indicated that they were confident that liaising with psychologists and getting therapy were the most significant support one could get for psycho-social stressors and early signs of mental health challenges. All participants indicated that they used Indima Yethu's six-step approach—"reach out, offer emotional support; offer affirmations and appraisal; offer informational support, offer instrumental support and share points of view" in helping people.

### *2.6.3 Outcome of Indima Yethu's six-step approach*

Items that fell within theme four focused on specific aspects of Indima Yethu's 13-week training resources which emphasized "self-concept, mentoring at least one person in their community (post training) and enabling peer access to social support through a six-step approach - 'reach out, offer emotional support; offer affirmations and appraisal; offer informational support, offer instrumental support and share points of view" among others. All participants but 2.6% (n = 14) reported that aspects of the course offering such as practicing active and empathetic listening during week 9 were very favorable. Many participants (98.7%, n = 541) indicated that taking the course helped them in finding their voice via blogging, defining what success and peace meant to them, taking baby steps toward it, and celebrating themselves. 52.7% (n = 289) of those who found the program very favorable indicated that they engaged in at least 30 minutes of moderate physical activity on most days of the week, journaling and telling instructors how they felt before and after each practice, 24.6% (n = 135) journaled but did not engage in any physical activity, and 22.6% (n = 124) did not journal nor engage in physical activity but reported observing their breath for 10 minutes each day and conducting energy mapping by observing when they were most productive each day and doing one little thing that pushed them out of their comfort zone.

98.7% (n = 541) of the participants who reported that the programs were very favorable indicated that the most positive aspects of were those that involved supporting their peers, pairing up with an established accountability partner to help them along the journey of achieving their set goals, practicing self-expression and coherence through daily journaling, identifying key areas of development related to career, academics, spirituality, and relationships and working on them, enlisting the support of family and friends in answering questions on self-awareness using a weekly prompt that was provided by Indima Yethu. The few participants (1.3%, n = 7) who found the program less favorable indicated the negative aspects were those that involved setting personal short- and long-term goals, and pairing up with an accountability partner who will hold them accountable. They reported that it put further strain on their mental health and did not help. **Table 2** presents examples and summaries of statements from participants.

## 2.7 Discussion

This study examines the effectiveness of a youth-focused Mental Health First Aid training program, within the context of an adapted adolescent guideline implemented by a nongovernmental organization in the Western Cape province of South Africa. It presents a preliminary attempt at building an evidence base for MHFA in South Africa by assessing the perceived impact on individuals who underwent training. The sample included young people between the age of 18 and 35 years who are resident in the Western Cape. Overall, the study findings indicate that MHFA is emerging in South Africa as a protective factor. Preliminary evaluation indicates wide acceptance

| Theme | Example statements |
|---|---|
| *Utilization of Knowledge* | We Black people do not like going for therapy and the older generation dismiss us as lazy when we complain but since I took this course, I have been able to encourage my cousins and I wish it could be translated it into Isizulu for my mom and aunties aunties. |
| | In all honesty, I live with extended family members who use alcohol to numb their pain but I used some of my knowledge to encourage them to seek help for their trauma. |
| | My living situation has been very volatile due to older siblings who are dealing with relationship issues and transferring aggression on others, but after taking the course, I have learned to listen non-judgmentally and give reassurance. |
| | Since I took the course, I have been the strong one for my family through all the losses we suffered during COVID-19. I have been listening to them and encouraging therapy. |
| | Since the day my grandmother started getting sick and even now, I have been the one facing it all, fighting it all through the help of ALGEE, to help encourage self-help support for my family. |
| | The course has helped me to the point where even my mother tells me things because she knows I will not judge her. |
| *Change in helping behavior* | Black communities see this as a taboo when one is suffering from mental health, and we are either told we sick and we need prayers. I think that what really draws people who suffer from it to commit suicide. Taking the YMHFA course helped me to recognize and adopt a more tolerant attitude toward mentally ill people. I am now comfortable talking to and helping them. |
| | I never liked the idea of being friends with or working with someone with a mental health problem, but ALGEE has helped me in starting conversations about how they can get help. |
| | I come from a community where people pray about mental illness or see a spiritualist who oftentimes tells them that it is a sign of spiritual calling. The course taught me a six-step approach I can use in persuading them to get help. |
| | To be honest, I used to be afraid of mentally ill people and thought they should be excluded, but now I know that no one is Immune to stressors. I mean, people can always get help if we apply the right strategies by educating them, not judging and referring them for professional help. This is humanity to me |
| Self-confidence | they began with an "asset mapping" instead of "needs analysis" in their course and that really helped us in learning about what is important to young people when it comes to applying ALGEE or making referrals. |
| | I think people with mental illness also value being involved in meaningful things that they also enjoy, including educational achievement, material wellbeing, housing, career success, and positive relationships. |
| | Indima Yethu's training enlightened me about self-consciousness, self-concept, and self-definition which also helped me in setting healthy boundaries and dealing with the stigma attached to having schizophrenia. People used to call me "schizo" but I am Now able to talk about my experience more openly and help others. |
| | Apart from the ALGEE plan, I benefited mostly from the mobile application and the breathing exercises which I've taught my family. It connects me to my higher self and grounds me. |
| | The course taught me a lot about myself and that has changed how I talk to people within my circle. I have referred over 20 people from my class for therapy since I completed the training and I am now working with primary schools. |

**Table 2.**
*Statements from participants showing broad spectrums and themes of MHFA impact.*

which corresponds with findings from a systematic review [31], of mostly quantitative studies which found that MHFA is an effective intervention for trainees exposed to the curriculum. They also indicated that the largest effect sizes were found for the knowledge and confidence outcomes, while "attitude and behavior-only" effect sizes were within the small range.

Participants in the current study indicated positive outcomes for MHFA training for them and their friends and family. Majority of the participants indicated that acquiring new information about mental health during their training changed their perception of mental illness and strengthened their confidence in supporting other people within their social network. Even though most of the samples are social science majors who did not participate through a compulsory university-based program, they reported using the knowledge gained to support their friends at school. Statements from participants suggested that adapted and culturally appropriate MHFA training guidelines for young people de-centered neediness and a token system which made communities heavily dependent on specialist services. Within this context, they noted that MHFA focused on identifying, building, and utilizing existing social capital capacities which contributed to improving the health of their communities.

In addition, the majority of the participants noted that YMHFA did not only connect people to others but helped in reconnecting them with their higher self and humanity. These findings strongly suggest that MHFA can be situated within a broader asset-based approach to mental health education. There is evidence of favorable outcomes such as new knowledge and de-stigmatization due to the inclusion of specific youth-friendly information and emphasis on social capital. Within the general pattern among the sample, findings suggest that MHFA is a protective factor which could potentially act at several different levels, including the individual, the family, the community, the structural, and the population levels when implemented in a culturally appropriate manner. Findings indicate that the observed positive changes in behavior and attitudes after MHFA training point to the role of effective health communication strategies in influencing intervention outcomes.

Due to the historical trajectories of South Africa, its long history of racial and economic inequality appears to have significantly influenced perceptions of mental illness among vulnerable social groups and access to coping resources that could protect or mitigate the impact of stressors as well as provide a buffer against risks. Since the end of apartheid, the new democratic government has struggled to sustain inclusive policies despite introducing social welfare packages for historically marginalized groups.

Reflecting on what is working well within a particular social group so that it can be included in training guidelines, considering what makes them strong or healthy as well as including other culturally appropriate items that make them more able to cope in times of stress, as the current study indicates, appears to increase positive outcomes for MHFA.

There was general satisfaction with the implementation of the 13-week program by Indima Yethu among those surveyed due to their emphasis on social determinants of general wellbeing and considerations for concepts, language, and priorities for various cultures and settings. To the majority of participants, the changes in their behavior stemmed from the cultural competence of the course and instructors which helped them and their loved ones in navigating relationships with professional service providers. There was evidence among all respondents of including information that addressed physical barriers to access, such as the sentinel mobile app which made referrals easier by connecting individuals to first responders. Based on surveys and

FGD data, participants felt that one of the most favorable aspects of the ALGEE training program was individuation, which made them aware of their specific stereotypes and biases against themselves and others.

## 3. Conclusion

This study examined the effectiveness of MHFA within the context of its growing popularity post-pandemic, and in particular, within regions without access to professional resources such as South Africa. Participants who had lived experiences of mental illness reported a higher satisfaction with the MHFA training due to their "embodied experiences and their desire to be understood by friends and family. As noted in the literature review, some existing body of work has shown that while MHFA had positive impacts on participants, it was more impactful on high-risk populations. In contrast to previous studies, the sample for the current research included individuals who had been diagnosed with and have experienced a particular mental illness and have lived with the 'stigma' of being misunderstood and misjudged by society (which is further reinforced by other participants who had not experienced mental illness of any kind, noting stigmatization and lack of empathy and support for youth living with mental illness. I believe that the positive feedback from participants is directly related to the emphasis on mindfulness, social capital, self-concept and the management of 'embodied experiences" in the course content.

This study suggests that MHFA plays a significant role in mental wellbeing management, health literacy, and de-stigmatization of mental health. Based on analysis of course content, focused group discussions, and direct observation, I conclude that four factors contributed to the overwhelming satisfaction experienced by participants: (1) the utilization of peer tutors in administering the training; (2) the inclusion of mental models and centering their agency in training content; (3) the availability of peer mentors and a mobile application which makes referral and access to professional intervention easy; and (4) the inclusion of friends and family as accountability partners.

To summarize, MHFA has the potential for positive outcomes when culturally and linguistically adapted. For example, within a global context, Black Africans, young people, females, the LGBT community, and others from marginalized social groups have a higher risk of mental illness, poor access to professional services, and acceptability-related challenges when the services are available; within most capitalist countries, this social group also suffers disproportionately more than others but are less likely to access MHFA, particularly, when such services lack cultural competence [32]. At the same time, while most MHFA training programs target vulnerable populations, some of the programs rarely reach them due to the exclusive focus on medicalization and specialized services [33]. The implication is that they tend to ignore such training [34]. The impact of cultural incompetence in the implementation of MHFA has had a significant effect on vulnerable individuals attempting to access mental health information or education through the public sector in imperialist states. This has implications for health outcomes over a life course.

The present study excluded most predictors of outcomes and changes in attitudes such as gender, age, and other measurable variables. The study also made no attempt at exploring the relationship between most variables and standard deviation. These have implications for future research. Further research is needed to cover these obvious limitations of the present study. In future research endeavors, caution must be applied in utilizing the result of this study to assess racial, gender, or SES-related disparities in

MHFA effectiveness. Future research should consider the impact and relationship of gender and education on identified outcomes in the current study. Existing patterns from positive MHFA training outcomes in the global north suggest that most MHFA trainees are more likely to be female, employed in care jobs that involve working with people, middle-aged than young, or males, and these measures matter.

## Notes/thanks/other declarations

NA.

## Author details

Chinwe Christopher Obuaku-Igwe
Department of Sociology, University of the Western Cape, South Africa

*Address all correspondence to: cobuaku@uwc.ac.za

## References

[1] Girgis K. Teen mental health first aid in the United States: A pilot study. In: Society for Prevention Research 28th Annual Meeting. SPR. Available from: https://spr.confex.com/spr/spr2020/meetingapp.cgi/Paper/29378 [Accessed: 23 October 2022]

[2] Davies EB, Beever E, Glazebrook C. A pilot randomized controlled study of the mental health first aid eLearning course with UK medical students. BMC Medical Education. 2018;**18**(1):1-2

[3] Drinkwater C, Wildman J, Moffatt S. Social prescribing. BMJ. 2019;**28**:364

[4] Sartore GM, Kelly B, Stain HJ, Fuller J, Fragar L, Tonna A. Improving mental health capacity in rural communities: Mental health first aid delivery in drought affected rural New South Wales. Australian Journal of Rural Health. 2008;**16**(5):313-318

[5] Mantzios M, Cook A, Egan H. Mental health first aid embedment within undergraduate psychology curriculums: An opportunity of applied experience for psychology students and for enhancing mental health care in higher education institutions. Higher Education Pedagogies. 2019;**4**(1):307-310

[6] Kitchener BA, Jorm AF. Mental Health First Aid: An international programme for early intervention. Early Intervention in Psychiatry. 2008;**2**(1):55-61

[7] Hadlaczky G, Hökby S, Mkrtchian A, Carli V, Wasserman D. Mental Health First Aid is an effective public health intervention for improving knowledge, attitudes, and behaviour: A meta-analysis. International Review of Psychiatry. 2014;**26**(4):467-475

[8] Jorm AF, Kitchener BA, Reavley NJ. Mental health first aid training: Lessons learned from the global spread of a community education program. World Psychiatry. 2019;**18**(2):142

[9] Mental Health First Aid International. Available from: https://mhfa.com.au/

[10] Jorm AF, Kitchener BA. Noting a landmark achievement: Mental health first aid training reaches 1% of Australian adults. Australian & New Zealand Journal of Psychiatry. 2011;**45**(10):808

[11] Sim T, Wang A. Contextualization of psychological first aid: An integrative literature review. Journal of Nursing Scholarship. 2021;**53**(2):189-197

[12] Ng SH, Tan NJ, Luo Y, Goh WS, Ho R, Ho CS. A systematic review of youth and teen mental health first aid: Improving adolescent mental health. Journal of Adolescent Health. 2021;**69**(2):199-210

[13] El-Den S, Moles R, Choong HJ, O'Reilly C. Mental Health First Aid training and assessment among university students: A systematic review. Journal of the American Pharmacists Association. 2020;**60**(5):e81-e95

[14] Costa TF, Sampaio FM, da Cruz Sequeira CA, Ribeiro IM, de Oliveira Parola VS. Mental health first aid programs: A scoping review protocol. JBI Evidence Synthesis. 2020;**18**(9):2011-2017

[15] Hart LM, Jorm AF, Paxton SJ, Cvetkovski S. Mental health first aid guidelines: An evaluation of impact following download from the World Wide Web. Early Intervention in Psychiatry. 2012;**6**(4):399-406

[16] Obuaku-Igwe C. 'Umuntu ngumuntu ngabantu'(a person is a person because of other people): Reflections on student's experiences of social isolation and the impact of a peer to peer mental health support group during covid-19 lockdown in South Africa. Youth Voice Journal. 2020;**2020**:58-71

[17] Hakulinen C, Elovainio M, Arffman M, Lumme S, Pirkola S, Keskimäki I, et al. Mental disorders and long-term labour market outcomes: Nationwide cohort study of 2,055,720 individuals. Acta Psychiatrica Scandinavica. 2019;**140**(4):371-381

[18] Mendenhall AN, Jackson SC, Hase S. Mental Health First Aid USA in a rural community: Perceived impact on knowledge, attitudes, and behavior. Social Work in Mental Health. 2022;**11**(6):563-577

[19] Noltemeyer A, Huang H, Meehan C, Jordan E, Morio K, Shaw K, et al. Youth mental health first aid: Initial outcomes of a statewide rollout in Ohio. Journal of Applied School Psychology. 2020;**36**(1):1-9

[20] Mental Health First Aid International. Available from:https://mhfainternational.org/international-mental-health-first-aid-programs/

[21] Colucci E, Kelly CM, Minas H, Jorm AF, Chatterjee S. Mental health first aid guidelines for helping a suicidal person: A Delphi consensus study in India. International Journal of mental health Systems. 2010;**4**(1):1-8

[22] Davies T, Roomaney R, Lund C, Sorsdahl K. Evaluation of an advocacy programme for mental health care users in South Africa: A mixed methods study. Community Mental Health Journal. 2022;**58**(4):720-728

[23] Saxena S, Thornicroft G, Knapp M, Whiteford H. Resources for mental health: Scarcity, inequity, and inefficiency. The Lancet. 2007;**370**(9590):878-889

[24] Kitchener B, Form A. Mental health first aid training: Review of evaluation studies. Australian & New Zealand Journal of Psychiatry. 2006;**40**(1):6-8. DOI: 10.1080/j.1440-1614.2006.01735.x

[25] Solmi M, Radua J, Olivola M, Croce E, Soardo L, Salazar de Pablo G, et al. Age at onset of mental disorders worldwide: Large-scale meta-analysis of 192 epidemiological studies. Molecular Psychiatry. 2022;**27**(1):281-295

[26] South African Federation for Mental Health (SAFM). Available from: https://www.safmh.org.za/wp-content/uploads/2020/09/SAFMH-Annual-Report-2018-2019.pdf

[27] Dworzanowski-Venter B. Is it time for a tele counselling revolution in South Africa? Exploring the views of clients and mental health professionals in the SADAG online community. Mental Health Matters. 2020;7(4):31-34

[28] Chevalier JM, Buckles DJ. Participatory Action Research: Theory and Methods for Engaged Inquiry. Routledge; 2019. Available from: https://www.tandfonline.com/doi/full/10.31887/DCNS.2009.11.1/krmerikangas [Accessed: 23 October 2022]

[29] Braun V, Clarke V. What can "thematic analysis" offer health and wellbeing researchers? International Journal of Qualitative Studies on Health and Well-being. 2014;**9**(1):26152

[30] Auerbach C, Silverstein LB. Qualitative Data: An Introduction to Coding and Analysis. NYU Press; 2003. Available from: https://www.safmh.org/

wp-content/uploads/2020/09/SAFMH-Annual-Report-2018-2019.pdf [Accessed: 23 October 2022]

[31] Maslowski AK, LaCaille RA, LaCaille LJ, Reich CM, Klingner J. Effectiveness of mental health first aid: A meta-analysis. Mental Health Review Journal. 2019;**7**(4):31-34. DOI: 10.10520/ejc-menhm-v7-n4-a10

[32] Costa TF, Sampaio FM, Sequeira CA, Ribeiro IM, Parola VS. Review of mental health first aid programs. Western Journal of Nursing Research. 2021;**43**(12):1146-1156

[33] DeFehr JN. Inventing mental health first aid: The problem of psychocentrism. Studies in Social Justice. 2016;**10**(1):18-35

[34] Jetten P. Developing empathy in school staff through emotional first aid. British Journal of School Nursing. 2011;**6**(7):353-355

Chapter 5

# Mental Health Conditions and Exercise

*Priscila Marconcin, Élvio Rúbio Gouveia, Marcelo de Maio Nascimento, Gerson Ferrari and Adilson Marques*

## Abstract

Mental health conditions are a major public health issue affecting many people worldwide. Evidence suggests that physical activity and exercise can prevent and treat mental health conditions, especially depression and anxiety. Several mechanisms are involved in the relationship between mental health conditions and exercise, from neurobiological to behavioural mechanisms. This chapter intends to explain the main mechanisms that explain that interaction and present recent evidence from studies that analyse the effects of exercise on mental health outcomes. It also highlights the principles of physical exercise (frequency, intensity, volume, and type) and how they can influence the main outcomes of mental health. Engaging in regular physical activity may prevent the onset of different mental health disorders. Also, evidence shows that exercise diminishes depressive symptoms. This chapter is indicated for health professionals who wish to have a broad view of the relationship between exercise and mental health. This knowledge can be valuable in designing public interventions that aim to treat mental disorders and optimise mental health.

**Keywords:** depression, anxiety, lifestyle, physical activity, mental health conditions

## 1. Introduction

Mental health is a multidimensional construct comprising emotional, psychological, and social dimensions of well-being [1]. In 1948, the World Health Organization stated that health is a complete physical, mental, and social well-being and not merely the absence of disease or infirmity. Although so many years have passed, many sectors of society continue to neglect mental health. There is still a stigma about mental health, which causes prejudice about the person suffering from a mental health disorder. Mental health disorders affect relationships with others, education, and work opportunities [2]. People with severe mental disorders are at the most risk of poverty and unemployment [3].

Mental health conditions are a global issue that increasingly affects people worldwide. It is estimated that one in every eight people in the world lives with a mental disorder [4]. Mental health conditions impact other health outcomes, including cardiovascular disease [5], premature death, and all-cause mortality [6]. Mental disorders account for 32.4% of years lived with disability (YLDs) and 13% of disability-adjusted life-years (DALYs) [7]. Major depressive disorder explained 16 million suicide DALYs and almost 4 million ischemic heart disease DALYs [2]. Also, mental health causes global and national economic loss, and depression and anxiety disorders cost the global economy US$ 1 trillion annually. More than half of the global economic burden attributable to non-communicable disease are from mental ill-health [8].

## 2. Deal with mental health conditions

In response to the impact caused by mental health conditions, the World Health Organization Mental Health Action Plan (2013–2030) aims to focus on four major objectives "more effective leadership and governance for mental health; the provision of comprehensive, integrated mental health and social care services in community-based settings; implementation of strategies for promotion and prevention; and strengthened information systems, evidence and research". This is a great effort to improve mental health, but much more needs to be done, especially considering low- and middle-income countries [9]. In general, mental health conditions can be treated at a relatively low cost; however, the gap between people needing care and those with access to care remains substantial.

Each mental health condition needs special attention to choose the best available treatment. Evidence has shown that lifestyle factors (physical activity, diet, tobacco smoking, and sleep) influence different psychiatric conditions. A meta-review concerning the role of modifiable lifestyle factors in preventing and treating mental disorders confirms that physical activity has a protective role in reducing the risk for certain mental disorders [10]. Physical activity provides effective adjunctive treatment for depression, anxiety and stress-related disorders, psychotic disorders, and attention-deficit/hyperactivity disorder (ADHD) [10]. Poor sleep has a causal role in bipolar disorder, and sleep disturbances have been found to significantly heighten the risk of suicidal behaviour in people with mental illness [10]. Smoking is associated with a heightened prospective risk of mental disorders, earlier age of onset, and adverse outcomes in those living with mental illness [10]. The causal effects of diet on common and severe mental conditions are less clear.

It is well recognised the effects of physical activity and exercise (structured physical activity) on several health outcomes, such as improvements in longevity, bone mineral density, cardiovascular risk factor, aerobic fitness, muscular strength and endurance, diabetes mellitus, obesity, some types of cancers, osteoporosis, and mental health [11]. Therefore, it is important to understand the association between physical activity and mental health conditions.

## 3. Mechanism that explains the association between exercise and mental health

Several mechanisms are involved in the association between exercise and mental health, from neurobiological to behavioural mechanisms and the integration of inter-related behavioural and neurobehavioral domains [12].

### 3.1 Inflammation

Exploring the neurobiological pathway through which exercise impacts mental health is needed. One potential biological mechanism is inflammation-related factors (IRFs), which have been linked with a broad range of psychiatric disorders [13]. The immune system moderates inflammation through several signalling pathways, particularly proteins like pro- and anti-inflammatory factors. Changes in some IRFs have been intensively studied and reviewed with psychiatric disorders, such as post-traumatic stress disorder (PTSD) [14], anxiety-based disorders [15], and autism spectrum disorder [16].

One possible explanation of increased inflammation is via activation of the stress response and central and peripheral immune cells to release cytokines [15]. Another explanation is that dysregulation of the stress axis in the face of increased sympathetic tone and decreased parasympathetic activity could further augment inflammation and consequently increase anxiety symptoms, affecting brain regions such as the prefrontal cortex, insula, amygdala, and hippocampus [15]. Also, some studies have shown an association between inflammatory markers and depressive symptoms, including fatigue, impaired sleep, and cognitive dysfunction [17].

Inflammation and neuropsychiatric disorders are possibly bidirectional, as occurs with depression. Depression facilitates inflammatory reactions, and inflammation promotes depression and other neuropsychiatric disorders [18]. A pharmacological meta-analysis study involving 2370 participants aimed to examine the potential role of cytokines in the treatment of depression showed a significant antidepressant effect of anti-cytokine treatment compared with placebo. The anti-TNF drug was the most commonly studied [19]. Some studies explained the pathways by which cytokines contribute to mental disorders: cytokines access the brain and interact with virtually every pathophysiologic domain relevant to mental illness, such as neurotransmitter metabolism, neuroendocrine function, and neural plasticity [20]. Exercise could create an anti-inflammatory environment and reduce the serum level of leptin and fibroblast growth factors (FGF) [21]. IL-10, produced by exercise, acts as an anti-inflammatory cytokine and is stimulated by the release of adrenaline and cortisol from the adrenal gland, reducing the release of proinflammatory cytokines in the hippocampus [22]. Therefore, inflammation could be a suitable biomarker for psychiatric disorders and help improve the accuracy of diagnosis and treatment of several psychiatric disorders.

### 3.2 Neuroplasticity

Neuroplasticity is the brain's ability to modify, change and adapt structure and function throughout life in response to experience. It is highly influenced by physical activity [12]. The increased neuroplastic capacity explains the mental health benefits of various somatic psychiatric treatments, such as selective serotonin reuptake inhibitors and trans-magnetic stimulation [12].

Several systemic factors, modifiable through exercise training, must be present to facilitate neuroplastic changes. Two essential factors include neurotrophins and low neuroinflammation. Neurotrophic growth factors increase with exercise and are linked to neuroplasticity, including modulation of brain-derived neurotrophic factor (BDNF), vascular endothelial growth factor (VEGF), and insulin-like growth factor 1 (IGF-1) [12]. Studies have shown that exercise increases BDNF production in the population with and without depression [23]. BDNF plays an important role in regulating synapse plasticity, affecting serotonin production in the hippocampus [23], and consequently impacts depressive symptoms. Also, exercise-enhancing VEGF and changing the vascular microenvironment were conducive to delivering oxygen-optimising neurogenesis [24].

### 3.3 Monoamines neurotransmitters (serotonin, norepinephrine, and dopamine)

Serotonin, norepinephrine, and dopamine are all monoamine neurotransmitters that modulate our mood. Depression has been consistently associated with impaired monoaminergic neurotransmission [25].

The cytokines can influence the synthesis, release, and reuptake of neurotransmitters [26]. Exercise may also influence depression by elevating the levels of endorphins and monoamines and regulating the hypothalamic-pituitary-adrenal axis.

### 3.4 Behavioural mechanism: the role of self-esteem and self-efficacy

Several aspects of the physical activity experience should be considered, such as enjoyment, mastery of skills/goals, autonomous motivation, social interaction, self-efficacy, self-esteem, and sense of belonging.

Exercise can promote several behavioural changes and may lead to a sense of mastery [27]. The activity-based perception of physical strength and flexibility is associated with increased physical self-esteem and, consequently, global self-esteem [28].

Self-efficacy is another important construct to better understand the relationship between exercise and mental health. Self-efficacy is an "individual's confidence in their ability to achieve specific, personally significant goals" [29]. Greater engagement in an exercise program has been shown to increase exercise self-efficacy [30] and improve self-image [31]. Self-esteem and self-efficacy mechanisms may explain the association between physical activity and depressive symptomatology [28].

Another important factor is the social interaction that the exercise can provide when performed as a group or just outdoors and is an important mediator of the association between exercise and depression, especially among older adults [32].

## 4. Physical activity guidelines for mental health conditions

The most recent physical activity guidelines from World Health Organization, in 2020, highlight the positive effects of physical activity on mental health, specifically reducing symptoms of anxiety and depression [33]. These recommendation covers subgroups, such as children and adolescents, adults, older adults, pregnant and postpartum women, adults and older adults with chronic conditions, children and adolescent, and adults living with disability, but did not include a specific recommendation to common mental illness, such as anxiety and depression.

The global recommendations suggest that adults should participate in at least 150–300 min of moderate-intensity aerobic physical activity or at least 75–150 min of vigorous-intensity aerobic physical activity per week and for additional health benefits on at least 2 days a week of muscle-strengthening activities at the moderate or greater intensity that involver all major muscle groups [33].

## 5. Physical activity and exercise for mental benefits

Several meta-analytic studies have investigated the association and the impact of physical activity on mental health outcomes. The results vary in efficacy degrees depending on methodological considerations, including study quality and duration [34].

Meta-analyses of prospective cohort studies have found that physical activity had a protective effect against the emergence of depression [35]. Also, physical activity protects against anxiety symptoms [36]. The association seems to be proportional since a higher level of physical fitness was associated with a lower onset of mental health problems [35]. In addition, sedentary behaviour is associated with an increased risk of depression [37] and anxiety [38].

Exercise exerts a causal influence on mental health disorders since exercise has a significant antidepressant effect in people with depression (including major depressive disorder) [39] and could improve anxiety symptoms in people with a current diagnosis of anxiety or stress-related disorders [40]. The antidepressant effect of aerobic exercise interventions was examined in a meta-analysis study and showed a significantly large effect [41]. The analysis revealed comparable effects across various settings and delivery formats, regardless of symptom severity in both outpatients and inpatients.

Furthermore, we can look forward and analyse the association between cardiorespiratory fitness (CRF) and common mental disorders. CRF captures broad physical activity trends with one discrete test using objective, clearly defined markers, such as oxygen consumption. The studies found that low and medium CRF is associated with an increased risk of common mental health disorders, namely depression [42] and anxiety [43].

Beyond cardiorespiratory fitness, muscle strength has also been associated with mental disorders. Increased hand grip strength may be associated with lower odds of developing generalised anxiety disorder [44]. Hand grip strength has been considered an important predictor of depressive symptoms in middle-aged and older adults [45].

Although several studies have demonstrated that physical activity can be used to prevent and treat common mental health disorders, most of the evidence assessed physical activity in general without analysing a dose-response of exercise, neither intensity, type, or other important aspects of exercise prescription.

### 5.1 Dose-response of the association between exercise and mental health functioning

Incremental increases in cardiorespiratory fitness are associated with proportional decreases in the risk of new-onset common mental health disorders, indicating a dose-response relationship between exercise and mental health disorders [43]. A national population-based study reveals that a minimal level of at least 20 min per week of physical activity guarantees mental health benefits. However, dose-response patterns demonstrated greater risk reduction for activity at a higher volume and intensity [46].

Meta-analyses of prospective cohort studies reveal that completing 150 min/week of moderate-vigorous physical activity reduces the risk of developing depression by about 22% [35]. However, low levels of physical activity (e.g., walking <150 min/week) can prevent future depression [47].

Exercise duration significantly moderates the effect of endurance intervention on depressive symptoms, and an extended exercise duration strengthens the antidepressant effect of endurance exercise interventions [48].

Regarding the bouts of exercise, a systematic review showed that short bouts (10–15 min) of physical activity had a significant effect on reducing stress and depressive symptoms and improving self-esteem among adults without mental health conditions [49].

Considering multiple dose-response curves of exercise regarding different health outcomes [50], no consensus about the optimal dose of physical activity to prevent or treat mental health was founded. For an increment of physical activity for the general population with mental health conditions, the World Health Organization policy seems to be a good way when proclaiming that "any movement counts" [33]. However, considering exercise prescriptions for each mental health condition, more systematic reviews of randomised controlled trials are needed to clarify the optimal dose response.

### 5.2 Intensity

A meta-analytical review concluded that increased exercise intensity of neuromuscular exercise strengthened the antidepressant effect among depressed adults [48]. Among older people with depression, moderate-intensity physical activity significantly affected depression [39]. Cross-sectional and prospective studies have demonstrated that moderate and vigorous physical activity intensity is associated with lower odds of depressive symptoms [51]. The best intensity to deal with depressive symptoms still needs more investigation.

A scoping review showed that there is not always a direct association between mental health and exercise duration/intensity [52]. In a study carried out with retired older adults, it was found that high-intensity physical activities had a negative impact on the perception of well-being [53]. A systematic review with meta-analysis of randomised controlled trials on sleep quality and insomnia in middle-aged women concluded that moderate levels of programmed exercise (aerobic exercise) indicated a positive effect on sleep quality. In contrast, low-intensity exercises did not reveal a significant effect [54]. These findings suggest that high-intensity exercise may not be the best strategy for well-being in the middle-aged and older adult population. A possible explanation is that this population tends to exercise to maintain physical fitness and also seek pro-social benefits, such as minimising isolation [55]. Consequently, practising exercises associated with social contact reflects positively on mental health [56]. Thus, moderate intensity seems to be the most useful measure of mental well-being.

### 5.3 Type of exercise

A meta-analysis including 1877 participants found that resistance exercise training was associated with a significant reduction in depressive symptoms, with a moderate-sized mean effect. However, a smaller reduction was observed when considering only trials with blinded allocation and assessment [57]. Similar anxiety results were found in another meta-analysis involving 922 participants, where resistance exercise training improves anxiety symptoms among healthy participants and participants with physical or mental disorders [58]. Combined aerobic moderate-vigorous physical activity and muscle-strengthening exercise were associated with the lowest likelihood of reporting depressive symptoms, analysed in a large population-based sample of adults (17,839 participants) [59].

Thus, when comparing aerobic exercise only and muscle-strengthening exercise only, no difference between modalities in reducing depressive symptoms was founded [42].

But adults who practice aerobic and muscle-strengthening physical activity combined had the lowest likelihood of depressive symptoms compared to those who adhere only to one exercise modality [59].

Other meta-analytical reviews revealed a moderate to large effect in favour of endurance exercise and a large effect in favour of neuromuscular exercise, compared to control conditions, to reduce depressive symptoms among depressed adults [48].

Among older adults with depression, a meta-analysis of randomised controlled trials found that mixed aerobic and anaerobic interventions significantly affected depression compared with the control group [39].

## 6. Conclusions

Mental health conditions represent a major impact on public health globally. People with mental conditions may be affected by several determinants related to physical, emotional, and social domains. This chapter aimed to elucidate alternatives to deal with mental conditions, highlighting the importance of physical activity and exercise. This underscores the importance of a multi-disciplinary approach to improve mental health that incorporates exercise as an essential part of treatment and prevention strategies. We present several mechanisms (neurobiological and behavioural) that are involved in the association between exercise and mental conditions. In line with the most recent guidelines, we expose the World Health Organization's general physical activity recommendation. Despite several evidence demonstrating the association between exercise and improvement in mental health outcomes, there is still a lack of clear guidelines on how to prescribe exercise based on the specific mental health condition and the principles of exercise (frequency, intensity, type, and duration). To finish this chapter, we present several pieces of evidence demonstrating the impact of exercise on mental health outcomes and explore the difference in dose response, intensity, and type of exercise.

The positive effects of physical activity and exercise on mental health are particularly relevant for public health interventions aimed at preventing and treating mental health disorders. We expected that this chapter would help future studies to fill some gaps in the literature and help health professionals to have a better understanding of the relationship between exercise and mental health outcomes.

## Conflict of interest

The authors declare no conflict of interest.

## Author details

Priscila Marconcin[1], Élvio Rúbio Gouveia[2], Marcelo de Maio Nascimento[3], Gerson Ferrari[4] and Adilson Marques[5]*

1 Instituto Piaget, Lisbon, Portugal

2 Universidade da Madeira, Funchal, Portugal

3 Federal University of Vale do São Francisco, Petrolina, Brazil

4 Universidad de Santiago de Chile, Santiago, Chile

5 Faculdade de Motricidade Humana, Universidade de Lisboa, Lisbon, Portugal

*Address all correspondence to: amarques@fmh.ulisboa.pt

## References

[1] Keyes CL. The mental health continuum: From languishing to flourishing in life. Journal of Health and Social Behavior. 2002;**43**(2):207-222

[2] Ferrari AJ, Charlson FJ, Norman RE, Patten SB, Freedman G, Murray CJL, et al. Burden of depressive disorders by country, sex, age, and year: Findings from the Global Burden of Disease Study 2010. PLoS Medicine. 2013;**10**(11):e1001547. DOI: 10.1371/journal.pmed.1001547

[3] Killaspy H, Harvey C, Brasier C, Brophy L, Ennals P, Fletcher J, et al. Community-based social interventions for people with severe mental illness: A systematic review and narrative synthesis of recent evidence. World Psychiatry. 2022;**21**(1):96-123. DOI: 10.1002/wps.20940

[4] GBD 2019 Mental Disorders Collaborators. Global, regional, and national burden of 12 mental disorders in 204 countries and territories, 1990-2019: A systematic analysis for the Global Burden of Disease Study 2019. Lancet Psychiatry. 2022;**9**(2):137-150. DOI: 10.1016/s2215-0366(21)00395-3

[5] Correll CU, Solmi M, Veronese N, Bortolato B, Rosson S, Santonastaso P, et al. Prevalence, incidence and mortality from cardiovascular disease in patients with pooled and specific severe mental illness: A large-scale meta-analysis of 3,211,768 patients and 113,383,368 controls. World Psychiatry. 2017;**16**(2):163-180. DOI: 10.1002/wps.20420

[6] Machado MO, Veronese N, Sanches M, Stubbs B, Koyanagi A, Thompson T, et al. The association of depression and all-cause and cause-specific mortality: An umbrella review of systematic reviews and meta-analyses. BMC Medicine. 2018;**16**(1):112. DOI: 10.1186/s12916-018-1101-z

[7] Vigo D, Thornicroft G, Atun R. Estimating the true global burden of mental illness. The Lancet Psychiatry. 2016;**3**(2):171-178. DOI: 10.1016/S2215-0366(15)00505-2

[8] Bloom DE, Cafiero E, Jané-Llopis E, Abrahams-Gessel S, Bloom LR, Fathima S, et al. The Global Economic Burden of Noncommunicable Diseases. Geneva: World Economic Forum; 2012

[9] Patel V, Saxena S, Lund C, Thornicroft G, Baingana F, Bolton P, et al. The Lancet Commission on global mental health and sustainable development. The Lancet. 2018;**392**(10157):1553-1598. DOI: 10.1016/S0140-6736(18)31612-X

[10] Firth J, Solmi M, Wootton RE, Vancampfort D, Schuch FB, Hoare E, et al. A meta-review of "lifestyle psychiatry": The role of exercise, smoking, diet and sleep in the prevention and treatment of mental disorders. World Psychiatry. 2020;**19**(3):360-380. DOI: 10.1002/wps.20773

[11] USDHHS. 2018 Physical Activity Guidelines Advisory Committee Scientific Report. Washington, DC: US Department of Health and Human Services; 2018

[12] Smith PJ, Merwin RM. The role of exercise in management of mental health disorders: An integrative review. Annual Review of Medicine. 2021;**72**:45-62

[13] Yuan N, Chen Y, Xia Y, Dai J, Liu C. Inflammation-related biomarkers in major psychiatric disorders:

A cross-disorder assessment of reproducibility and specificity in 43 meta-analyses. Translational Psychiatry. 2019;**9**(1):233. DOI: 10.1038/s41398-019-0570-y

[14] Gill JM, Saligan L, Woods S, Page G. PTSD is associated with an excess of inflammatory immune activities. Perspectives in Psychiatric Care. 2009;**45**(4):262-277. DOI: 10.1111/j.1744-6163.2009.00229.x

[15] Michopoulos V, Powers A, Gillespie CF, Ressler KJ, Jovanovic T. Inflammation in fear- and anxiety-based disorders: PTSD, GAD, and beyond. Neuropsychopharmacology. 2017;**42**(1):254-270. DOI: 10.1038/npp.2016.146

[16] Tonhajzerova I, Ondrejka I, Mestanik M, Mikolka P, Hrtanek I, Mestanikova A, et al. Inflammatory activity in autism spectrum disorder. Advances in Experimental Medicine and Biology. 2015;**861**:93-98. DOI: 10.1007/5584_2015_145

[17] Motivala SJ, Sarfatti A, Olmos L, Irwin MR. Inflammatory markers and sleep disturbance in major depression. Psychosomatic Medicine. 2005;**67**(2):187-194. DOI: 10.1097/01.psy.0000149259.72488.09

[18] Bauer ME, Teixeira AL. Inflammation in psychiatric disorders: What comes first? Annals of the New York Academy of Sciences. 2019;**1437**(1):57-67. DOI: 10.1111/nyas.13712

[19] Kappelmann N, Lewis G, Dantzer R, Jones PB, Khandaker GM. Antidepressant activity of anti-cytokine treatment: A systematic review and meta-analysis of clinical trials of chronic inflammatory conditions. Molecular Psychiatry. 2018;**23**(2):335-343. DOI: 10.1038/mp.2016.167

[20] Miller AH, Maletic V, Raison CL. Inflammation and its discontents: The role of cytokines in the pathophysiology of major depression. Biological Psychiatry. 2009;**65**(9):732-741. DOI: 10.1016/j.biopsych.2008.11.029

[21] Fedewa MV, Hathaway ED, Ward-Ritacco CL, Williams TD, Dobbs WC. The effect of chronic exercise training on leptin: A systematic review and meta-analysis of Randomized Controlled Trials. Sports Medicine. 2018;**48**(6):1437-1450. DOI: 10.1007/s40279-018-0897-1

[22] Moon HY, Kim SH, Yang YR, Song P, Yu HS, Park HG, et al. Macrophage migration inhibitory factor mediates the antidepressant actions of voluntary exercise. Proceedings of the National Academy of Sciences. 2012;**109**(32):13094-13099. DOI: 10.1073/pnas.1205535109

[23] Kurdi FN, Flora R. Physical exercise increased brain-derived neurotrophic factor in elderly population with depression. Open access Macedonian Journal of Medical Sciences. 2019;**7**(13):2057

[24] Morland C, Andersson KA, Haugen ØP, Hadzic A, Kleppa L, Gille A, et al. Exercise induces cerebral VEGF and angiogenesis via the lactate receptor HCAR1. Nature Communications. 2017;**8**(1):15557. DOI: 10.1038/ncomms15557

[25] Hamon M, Blier P. Monoamine neurocircuitry in depression and strategies for new treatments. Progress in Neuro-Psychopharmacology & Biological Psychiatry. 2013;**45**:54-63. DOI: 10.1016/j.pnpbp.2013.04.009

[26] Miller AH. Norman Cousins Lecture. Mechanisms of cytokine-induced behavioral changes: Psychoneuroimmunology at the

translational interface. Brain, Behavior, and Immunity. 2009;**23**(2):149-158. DOI: 10.1016/j.bbi.2008.08.006

[27] Gheysen F, Poppe L, DeSmet A, Swinnen S, Cardon G, de Bourdeaudhuij I, et al. Physical activity to improve cognition in older adults: Can physical activity programs enriched with cognitive challenges enhance the effects? A systematic review and meta-analysis. International Journal of Behavioral Nutrition and Physical Activity. 2018;**15**(1):63. DOI: 10.1186/s12966-018-0697-x

[28] Ryan MP. The antidepressant effects of physical activity: Mediating self-esteem and self-efficacy mechanisms. Psychology & Health. 2008;**23**(3):279-307. DOI: 10.1080/14768320601185502

[29] Bandura A. Self-efficacy. In: Ramachaudran VS, editor. Encyclopedia of Human Behavior. New York: Academic Press. pp. 71-81

[30] Olson EA, McAuley E. Impact of a brief intervention on self-regulation, self-efficacy and physical activity in older adults with type 2 diabetes. Journal of Behavioral Medicine. 2015;**38**(6):886-898. DOI: 10.1007/s10865-015-9660-3

[31] Berli C, Stadler G, Shrout PE, Bolger N, Scholz U. Mediators of physical activity adherence: Results from an action control intervention in couples. Annals of Behavioral Medicine. 2018;**52**(1):65-76

[32] Herbolsheimer F, Ungar N, Peter R. Why is social isolation among older adults associated with depressive symptoms? The mediating role of out-of-home physical activity. International Journal of Behavioral Medicine. 2018;**25**(6):649-657. DOI: 10.1007/s12529-018-9752-x

[33] World Health Organization. WHO Guidelines on Physical Activity and Sedentary Behaviour. Geneva: WHO; 2020

[34] Krogh J, Nordentoft M, Sterne JA, Lawlor DA. The effect of exercise in clinically depressed adults: Systematic review and meta-analysis of randomised controlled trials. The Journal of Clinical Psychiatry. 2011;**72**(4):529-538. DOI: 10.4088/JCP.08r04913blu

[35] Schuch FB, Vancampfort D, Firth J, Rosenbaum S, Ward PB, Silva ES, et al. Physical activity and incident depression: A meta-analysis of prospective cohort studies. The American Journal of Psychiatry. 2018;**175**(7):631-648. DOI: 10.1176/appi.ajp.2018.17111194

[36] Schuch FB, Stubbs B, Meyer J, Heissel A, Zech P, Vancampfort D, et al. Physical activity protects from incident anxiety: A meta-analysis of prospective cohort studies. Depression and Anxiety. 2019;**36**(9):846-858. DOI: 10.1002/da.22915

[37] Teychenne M, Ball K, Salmon J. Sedentary behavior and depression among adults: A review. International Journal of Behavioral Medicine. 2010;**17**(4):246-254. DOI: 10.1007/s12529-010-9075-z

[38] Teychenne M, Costigan SA, Parker K. The association between sedentary behaviour and risk of anxiety: A systematic review. BMC Public Health. 2015;**15**(1):513. DOI: 10.1186/s12889-015-1843-x

[39] Schuch FB, Vancampfort D, Richards J, Rosenbaum S, Ward PB, Stubbs B. Exercise as a treatment for depression: A meta-analysis adjusting for publication bias. Journal of Psychiatric Research. 2016;**77**:42-51. DOI: 10.1016/j.jpsychires.2016.02.023

[40] Stubbs B, Vancampfort D, Rosenbaum S, Firth J, Cosco T, Veronese N, et al. An examination of the anxiolytic effects of exercise for people with anxiety and stress-related disorders: A meta-analysis. Psychiatry Research. 2017;**249**:102-108. DOI: 10.1016/j.psychres.2016.12.020

[41] Morres ID, Hatzigeorgiadis A, Stathi A, Comoutos N, Arpin-Cribbie C, Krommidas C, et al. Aerobic exercise for adult patients with major depressive disorder in mental health services: A systematic review and meta-analysis. Depression and Anxiety. 2019;**36**(1):39-53. DOI: 10.1002/da.22842

[42] Schuch FB, Vancampfort D, Sui X, Rosenbaum S, Firth J, Richards J, et al. Are lower levels of cardiorespiratory fitness associated with incident depression? A systematic review of prospective cohort studies. Preventive Medicine. 2016;**93**:159-165. DOI: 10.1016/j.ypmed.2016.10.011

[43] Kandola A, Ashdown-Franks G, Stubbs B, Osborn DPJ, Hayes JF. The association between cardiorespiratory fitness and the incidence of common mental health disorders: A systematic review and meta-analysis. Journal of Affective Disorders. 2019;**257**:748-757. DOI: 10.1016/j.jad.2019.07.088

[44] Gordon BR, McDowell CP, Lyons M, Herring MP. Associations between grip strength and generalised anxiety disorder in older adults: Results from the Irish longitudinal study on ageing. Journal of Affective Disorders. 2019;**255**:136-141. DOI: 10.1016/j.jad.2019.05.043

[45] Marques A, Henriques-Neto D, Peralta M, Marconcin P, Gouveia ÉR, Ferrari G, et al. Exploring grip strength as a predictor of depression in middle-aged and older adults. Scientific Reports. 2021;**11**(1):15946. DOI: 10.1038/s41598-021-95566-7

[46] Hamer M, Stamatakis E, Steptoe A. Dose-response relationship between physical activity and mental health: The Scottish Health Survey. British Journal of Sports Medicine. 2009;**43**(14):1111-1114. DOI: 10.1136/bjsm.2008.046243

[47] Mammen G, Faulkner G. Physical activity and the prevention of depression: A systematic review of prospective studies. American Journal of Preventive Medicine. 2013;**45**(5):649-657. DOI: 10.1016/j.amepre.2013.08.001

[48] Nebiker L, Lichtenstein E, Minghetti A, Zahner L, Gerber M, Faude O, et al. Moderating effects of exercise duration and intensity in neuromuscular vs. Endurance exercise interventions for the treatment of depression: A meta-analytical review. Frontiers in Psychiatry. 2018;**9**:305. DOI: 10.3389/fpsyt.2018.00305

[49] Barr-Anderson DJ, AuYoung M, Whitt-Glover MC, Glenn BA, Yancey AK. Integration of short bouts of physical activity into organisational routine a systematic review of the literature. American Journal of Preventive Medicine. 2011;**40**(1):76-93. DOI: 10.1016/j.amepre.2010.09.033

[50] Warburton DE, Charlesworth S, Ivey A, Nettlefold L, Bredin SS. A systematic review of the evidence for Canada's Physical Activity Guidelines for Adults. International Journal of Behavioral Nutrition and Physical Activity. 2010;7:39. DOI: 10.1186/1479-5868-7-39

[51] Marques A, Bordado J, Peralta M, Gouveia ER, Tesler R, Demetriou Y, et al. Cross-sectional and prospective relationship between physical activity and depression symptoms. Scientific

Reports. 2020;**10**(1):16114. DOI: 10.1038/s41598-020-72987-4

[52] Kadariya S, Gautam R, Aro AR. Physical activity, mental health, and wellbeing among older adults in South and Southeast Asia: A scoping review. BioMed Research International. 2019;**2019**:6752182. DOI: 10.1155/2019/6752182

[53] Lee YJ, Hung WL. The relationship between exercise participation and well-being of the retired elderly. Aging & Mental Health. 2011;**15**(7):873-881. DOI: 10.1080/13607863.2011.569486

[54] Rubio-Arias J, Marín-Cascales E, Ramos-Campo DJ, Hernandez AV, Pérez-López FR. Effect of exercise on sleep quality and insomnia in middle-aged women: A systematic review and meta-analysis of randomised controlled trials. Maturitas. 2017;**100**:49-56. DOI: 10.1016/j.maturitas.2017.04.003

[55] Chekroud SR, Gueorguieva R, Zheutlin AB, Paulus M, Krumholz HM, Krystal JH, et al. association between physical exercise and mental health in 1·2 million individuals in the USA between 2011 and 2015: A cross-sectional study. Lancet Psychiatry. 2018;**5**(9):739-746. DOI: 10.1016/s2215-0366(18)30227-x

[56] Schuch FB, Vancampfort D. Physical activity, exercise, and mental disorders: It is time to move on. Trends in Psychiatry Psychotherapy. 2021;**43**(3):177-184. DOI: 10.47626/2237-6089-2021-0237

[57] Gordon BR, McDowell CP, Hallgren M, Meyer JD, Lyons M, Herring MP. Association of efficacy of resistance exercise training with depressive symptoms: Meta-analysis and Meta-regression Analysis of Randomised Clinical Trials. JAMA Psychiatry. 2018;**75**(6):566-576. DOI: 10.1001/jamapsychiatry.2018.0572

[58] Gordon BR, McDowell CP, Lyons M, Herring MP. The effects of resistance exercise training on anxiety: A meta-analysis and meta-regression analysis of Randomized Controlled Trials. Sports Medicine. 2017;**47**(12):2521-2532. DOI: 10.1007/s40279-017-0769-0

[59] Bennie JA, Teychenne MJ, De Cocker K, Biddle SJH. Associations between aerobic and muscle-strengthening exercise with depressive symptom severity among 17,839 U.S. adults. Preventive Medicine. 2019;**121**:121-127. DOI: 10.1016/j.ypmed.2019.02.022

Chapter 6

# Perspective Chapter: The Impact of COVID-19 on Mental Health – The Protective Role of Resilience and Capacity for Mentalizing

*Teodora Safiye, Medo Gutić, Ardea Milidrag, Milena Zlatanović and Branimir Radmanović*

## Abstract

The COVID-19 pandemic has caused enormous psychological impact worldwide, and represents an unprecedented threat to mental health. There are significant individual differences in adaptation to a stressful situation such as a pandemic, which depends on personality characteristics and psychological resources such as resilience and capacity for mentalizing. Research shows that a good capacity for mentalizing and resilience are a protective factors for mental health, which can be acquired through an appropriate education and training programs. The objective of this chapter is to summarize the extant literature reporting on mental health, ie. the prevalence of symptoms of depression, anxiety, and others forms of psychological distress during the COVID-19 pandemic. An additional objective is to identify the role of preventive factors: resilience and capacity for mentalizing, which are associated with mental health. Findings from the extensive scientific literature prove that the outbreak of the COVID-19 pandemic has increased the prevalence of mental health problems by a massive 25% worldwide and that resilience and good mental capacity play a significant role in reducing mental health disorders.

**Keywords:** mental health, COVID-19, resilience, capacity for mentalizing, depression, stress, fear

## 1. Introduction

At the end of 2019, a new type of previously unidentified coronavirus appeared in the Chinese city of Wuhan, then known as the novel coronavirus 2019, which was renamed SARS-CoV-2, severe acute respiratory syndrome coronavirus 2. The disease it causes is officially named Coronavirus Disease-2019 (COVID-19). The first cases of infection with this virus spread from animals to humans, presumably at the seafood market in the Chinese city of Wuhan, causing a terrible epidemic in many cities in China [1, 2]. Due to the growing rate of reporting cases in Chinese and international locations, on January 30, 2020, the WHO Emergency Committee declared a global health emergency [2].

To slow the spread of COVID-19 and prevent health systems from becoming overloaded, many countries around the world have implemented restrictions on population movement and complete or partial lockdowns, police-enforced curfew, strict travel bans and shutted borders [3]. All of this has affected the established way of human life and caused a major psychological impact on people around the world, posing a serious threat to mental health [3].

The severity of the COVID-19 pandemic poses a new challenge to mental health. The World Health Organization defines mental health as a state of well-being in which an individual achieves his potential, can cope with normal life stress, can work productively and is able to contribute to the community. The definition of mental health leads to the conclusion that it is more than just the absence of mental illness, ie that good functioning within one's own family, good relationships with other people and expressing life satisfaction are qualities of a person who is mentally healthy [4]. People with good mental health are often sad, sick, angry or unhappy, and that is part of a fully lived life for a human being. Nevertheless, mental health is often conceptualized as a purely positive impact, marked by a sense of happiness and a sense of having control over one's environment [4].

With the outbreak of COVID-19, people faced a series of situations that changed their lives, but also the lives of their loved ones. Closing in houses, distancing oneself from other people, death of close people and general uncertainty are situations to which people were not used until then [3, 5]. The continuing stress associated with a pandemic can have serious consequences for their mental health. Stress involves physiological and psychological reactions to stressors that come from the environment, and people very often have no control over these causes of stress [6].

Depression, anxiety, and stress have been identified as basic negative indicators of mental health and some of the major health problems, and research interest has focused on understanding their nature, causes, and treatments [7]. An individual's depression is characterized by experiences of dysphoria, hopelessness, devaluation of oneself and life as a whole, impoverishment of social life and anhedonia. Anxiety is a mental state characterized by a subjective experience of anxiety, a feeling of helplessness and a high level of arousal of the organism. Negative stress is a state of high arousal of the organism that occurs as a result of one or more threatening events, with strong negative emotions on the mental level [7]. People who are generally prone to anxiety, as a rule, often express symptoms of depression, and vice versa. Stress is also associated with depression and anxiety [7].

Studies assessing stress, anxiety and depression during quarantine caused by the spread of SARS-CoV-2 have revealed the presence of severe psychological distress and psychopathological factors and have shown that the COVID-19 pandemic is associated with very significant levels of stress, which in many cases could reach the threshold of clinical importance [8].

Further in the text of this book chapter, a more detailed review of the existing literature on mental health and associated factors during the COVID-19 pandemic will be reported, ie the prevalence of symptoms of depression, anxiety and other forms of psychological distress. After that, the roles of preventive factors related to mental health will be identified, with a focus on resilience and capacity for mentalizing.

## 2. COVID-19 pandemic and mental health disorders

The outbreak of the COVID-19 pandemic caused an increase in the prevalence of mental disorders by a massive 25%. The most common and important of these disorders are depression, anxiety and various types of psychological distress, which are described in more detail in this book chapter. In addition to the COVID-19 pandemic, multiple factors also caused a "pandemic of mental disorders", ie a massive increase in mental health problems.

One of the main explanations for the increase in mental health problems is the unprecedented multiple stress caused by the social isolation resulting from the pandemic. Related to this were limitations in people's ability to work, seek support from loved ones and engage in their communities, loneliness, fear of infection, suffering and death for themselves and loved ones, grief after bereavement, and financial worries. These are all stressors that lead to the fundamental mental problems of anxiety and depression. Among healthcare workers, who belong to a group particularly vulnerable to the COVID-19 pandemic, exhaustion and burnout syndrome have been main triggers for suicidal thoughts [3, 5].

### 2.1 COVID-19 pandemic and mental health status in the general population

Numerous studies on the mental health status of people around the world have been published during the COVID-19 pandemic, reporting on different rates of mental health problems. Some differences can be attributed to methodological issues such as different instruments for measuring mental health indicators such as depression, anxiety and distress, and the range of outcomes used, while other differences probably stemmed from cultural factors about discovering mental health problems [9].

A review of research literature from China, India, Nepal, Iran, Iraq, Japan, Nigeria, the United Kingdom, Italy and Spain showed that the average prevalence of depression in 14 studies with a sample size of 44,531 people was 33.7%, the prevalence of anxiety in 17 studies with a sample size of 63,439 was 31.9%, while stress rates in 5 studies with a total sample size of 9074 individuals were 29.6% [10].

When it comes to the results of research conducted in Europe, similar findings have been obtained. The first study in Serbia examining the mental health status of the general adult population found that of the 1057 participants in the study, 28.9% reported moderate to severe depression, 36.9% moderate to severe anxiety, and 38.1% moderate to severe symptoms of stress. Fear about COVID-19 news, feelings of helplessness, the likelihood of impending death, and the presence of COVID-19 symptoms were associated with higher levels of depression, anxiety, and stress. Current smoking status was associated with a higher risk of depression and stress. Higher socioeconomic status was significantly associated with lower levels of depression, anxiety and stress, while students had significantly higher levels of depression and stress [3].

Isolation, reduced social contacts, the duration of quarantine and restrictions, and significant changes in access to higher education in response to the global COVID-19 pandemic have played an important role in increasing negative emotional symptoms and stress in students. A study conducted on a sample of 338 students in Serbia during the state of emergency due to the COVID-19 pandemic examined the relationship between depression, anxiety, stress and procrastination [11]. The results showed that the average values of depression, anxiety and stress among students were significantly higher compared to the findings of research conducted on a sample of university students before the pandemic in Serbia, but also in other European countries [11].

The psychological impact of COVID-19 on the university community has also been demonstrated in research conducted in Spain, Greece and France. According to research conducted in Spain during the first weeks of the introduction of curfew due to the pandemic, students showed higher scores on the scales of depression, anxiety and stress, compared to the situation before the COVID-19 pandemic [12]. The authors, who conducted research in Greece during the state of emergency due to the COVID-19 pandemic, pointed to an increase in anxiety, depression and psychological distress in students compared to the time before the pandemic [13]. A cross-sectional study aimed at assessing the prevalence of anxiety and identifying anxiety-related factors among French students during the outbreak of COVID-19 found that of the 3936 students, 15.2% experienced moderate anxiety. Female gender and having relatives or acquaintances who were hospitalized for COVID-19 were major risk factors for anxiety [14].

Systematic review of three electronic databases (Google Scholar, PubMed and Medline), with 13 studies from different European countries that published data on the prevalence of anxiety, depression and stress in students, showed that the overall combined prevalence rate was 55% for anxiety, 63% for depression and 62% for stress [15]. A significant increase in anxiety, depression and stress has been identified among university students across Europe, but the long-term effect of this will need to be monitored. Governments, universities and other higher education service providers should take into account students' mental health and provide strategies to support their mental well-being [15].

A study examining mental health during the COVID-19 pandemic and key risk factors in the adult population in Croatia, on a nationally representative sample of 1201 participants, shows that 9.8% of respondents were at risk of adjustment disorders, 7.7% were at risk of developing depressive disorder, and 7.8% were at risk for anxiety disorder. In addition, 7.2% experienced high levels of stress. Key risk factors for specific negative mental health outcomes varied, but common predictive factors for some of the mental health problems included younger age, current health status, previous diagnosis of mental disorder, having an below-average income, and over-following COVID-19 news. Together, the key risk factors identified in this study indicate the need for public health interventions that address the mental health of the general population, but also for specific risk groups [16].

## 2.2 COVID-19 pandemic and mental health status in the population of healthcare workers

COVID-19 has a serious impact on the mental health of both the general population and healthcare workers who belong to a special risk group during a pandemic [3, 17]. The psychological impact of the outbreak of acute infections on health workers has caused significant concern to the government, the public and medical professionals. The psychological impact of COVID-19 on health workers working during a pandemic is an important consideration, as chronic exposure to stressors leads to burnout syndrome and various mental health problems [17].

One study on psychological distress, which included 958 health workers from the city of Wuhan in China, indicates that more than half of the respondents had symptoms related to depression and anxiety. Specifically, 54% of the total sample had symptoms of anxiety and 58% of depression, with the prevalence of stress being higher than previously detected in healthcare workers battling the SARS virus [18]. In the study which involved 1257 healthcare workers from China, of which 760 from Wuhan, 71.5% of respondents showed symptoms of stress, 44.6% anxiety, 50.4% depression and 34% insomnia. These symptoms were more severe in nurses, front-line staff, and those working in Wuhan, the epicenter of the COVID-19 pandemic outbreak [19]. Similar results have been found in European countries, such as Germany, where healthcare professionals, especially nurses, have reported a high prevalence of stress, emotional fatigue and depressive symptoms [20].

A study conducted in China found that healthcare workers at the frontline of the pandemic and who deal directly with patients confirmed or suspected of having COVID-19 have higher levels of various mental health problems than those working in regular clinical settings. In addition, these two groups had comparatively low rates of behavior seeking help and treatment for their mental health problems. Data from that study showed that the mental health of healthcare workers at the frontline is of particular concern. The rate of mental health problems, such as anxiety, depression and insomnia, has increased significantly among healthcare workers working on the front lines of the fight against COVID-19, compared to those without direct contact with COVID-19 [21].

Compared to non-frontline healthcare workers, frontline healthcare workers can be exposed to much greater physical and mental stress, which can contribute to a higher rate of mental health problems. For example, frontline healthcare workers had to be especially careful when working in respiratory units or infectious wards, ensuring that suspicious patients were identified in a timely manner and transferred to a particular hospital to reduce the risk of exposure to others [21]. These results showed poor mental health among healthcare workers at the frontline of the fight against COVID-19 [21], but contrary to expectations, no significantly higher rates of seeking help or treatment of mental health problems were observed among these individuals. The phenomenon that healthcare professionals have difficulty accepting and detecting emotions is not unique to the outbreak of the COVID-19 pandemic [22]. Emotional stress is common among hospital physicians, many of whom do not seek professional help or support from their colleagues because they either think they did not need it or are uncomfortable seeking help and are concerned about confidentiality [22]. These findings remind us that in the future, providers of psychological interventions should pay more attention to healthcare workers who have mental health problems.

Study examining healthcare workers before and during the outbreak of the COVID-19 pandemic [23], which included both those working on the front lines and those with unclear COVID-19 exposure, found that the incidence of anxiety, depression and insomnia increased over time. However, it is unclear whether the respondents were the same at both time points. During the outbreak of COVID-19, one in four healthcare professionals reported at least mild anxiety, depression or insomnia [23].

One meta-analysis showed that twenty-two studies reported one or more variables related to mental health problems in healthcare workers during the COVID-19 pandemic [24]. The most common risk factors correlated with an increased risk of mental health problems were exposure to patients with COVID-19, females [24] and concerns of health professionals that they would be infected with coronavirus [21, 24]. In three studies, concern that family members were infected was a risk factor [24]. When it comes to anxiety, data from 22 studies showed that the percentage of healthcare workers with anxiety ranged from 9 to 90% with a median of 24% [24]. For depression, there were data from 19 studies. The percentage of respondents with depression ranged from 5 to 51%, with a median of 21%. For sleep problems, there were data from six studies. The percentage of sleep problems ranged from 34 to 65%, with a median of 37%. For psychological distress, there were data from 13 studies. The percentage with distress ranged from 7 to 97%, with a median of 37% [24].

The aforementioned studies conducted around the world during the COVID-19 pandemic highlighted mental health problems and unmet needs of medical staff during the pandemic. There is an urgent need to provide further strategies to alleviate the mental health problems of health workers, and long-term monitoring of the mental health of health workers, both those at the first line and those at the secont line of the COVID-19 pandemic [21].

## 3. Protective factors of mental health during the COVID-19

In addition to COVID-19-related mental health risk factors, which mainly include the following: female gender and age under 40 [25–27], student status, unemployment, poor economic status, lower level of education and unemployment [3, 27–29], presence of chronic illness and history of medical or psychiatric illness [20, 30, 31], as well as frequent exposure to social media and news related to COVID-19 [3, 26, 32], and inadequate information about the virus [5, 33], several studies have also identified factors that protect individuals from symptoms of mental disorders during the COVID-19 pandemic. These factors associated with COVID-19 mainly include the timely dissemination of up-to-date and accurate health information regarding COVID-19 by the competent authorities [29], the active implementation of precautionary measures to reduce the risk of infection, such as frequent hand washing, wearing masks and less contact with people, [29], as well as more social support [34], and rest time during a pandemic [35].

Besides to these factors that are specific to the COVID-19 pandemic, it has been shown that psychological symptoms during a pandemic may be related to some personality traits, such as temperament, positive stress coping mehanisms [36, 37], secure and avoidant attachment styles [29, 37], resilience [33, 38–41], and capacity for mentalizing [42].

### 3.1 Resilience

There are significant individual differences in adapting to stressful situations such as the COVID-19 pandemic, which depends on personality characteristics and psychological resources, such as resilience. Previous studies have found that mental health during the pandemic has been associated with positive psychological traits such as psychological resilience [38, 39] and hope [40], and that resilience positively stabilizes mental health during the COVID-19 pandemic [41].

Interest in psychological resilience has increased in recent decades [43]. Numerous scientific disciplines deal with resilience, starting from psychiatry and psychology, through sociology to medicine, genetics and neuroscience. Nevertheless, by reviewing the existing literature and the definition of this term, the only consensus exists, and that is the question "how some people can endure discomfort without negative physical and psychological consequences" [44]. This is exactly how the simplest definition of the resilience construct can be formulated - as the ability of people to function well in difficult situations, that is, to cope with the stress that often accompanies them. Synonyms such as hardiness, resistance, psychoimmunity and toughness further clarify the qualities that resilience implies. Simply put, resilience implies successful adaptation and the ability to maintain or regenerate mental health despite obstacles [45]. In addition, it can be characterized as a process of evolution of positive attitudes and strategies [46], but also as an individual's ability to "go back to the old" [43, 47].

Multidisciplinarity in approaching this problem has made definitions change and evolve as scientific understanding and cognition changes.

When resilience is perceived as a personality trait, it refers to an individual's ability to return to a state of normal mental functioning after stressful or threatening events, without lasting negative consequences [43].

When resilience is defined as a complex capacity of an individual, then it is understood as the result of all protective factors that act to maintain or improve an individual's mental health after circumstances that may cause severe distress or mental trauma. These protective factors can be: 1) individual factors, such as e.g. ways of overcoming stress, cognitive capacity and strength of an individual's character, 2) factors arising from an individual's social network, such as e.g. emotional or material support provided by family or close friends, and 3) support from the wider community, such as support provided by government agencies, businesses, and social organizations [43, 48].

Previous studies have shown that resilience is negatively correlated with depression and anxiety [49–51]. Even before the COVID-19 pandemic, high resilience was cited as a complex trait that allows people to easily recover from a variety of difficulties, which can be acquired through an appropriate training program [52–54]. Resilience is also cited as a trait that can reduce the association between burnout syndrome and mental health difficulties, and which acts as a moderator as a moderator by alleviating the association between burnout syndrome and subjective well-being [48, 55, 56].

The results of a study examining the links between resilience, hope, preventive behavior, subjective well-being and mental health in 220 adults, in the early stages of the COVID-19 pandemic, showed that hope and resilience have significant direct effects on mental health and subjective well-being. Preventive behavior showed no significant effect on these two variables other than resilience. These results suggest that more attention needs to be paid to hope and resilience to develop and improve well-being and mental health in times of crisis [40].

Research has found that resilience characteristics are associated with lower levels of anxiety and depression symptoms [57] and that resilience has mediated the relationship between stress, anxiety and depression symptoms [58]. Generally speaking, people with a higher degree of resilience also have a higher degree of well-being, and a lower degree of depression, anxiety and negative self-evaluation [54, 59].

### 3.2 Capacity for mentalizing

Good capacity for mentalizing is considered to play a preventive role in maintaining mental health. Mentalizing is a form of imaginative mental activity that consists of interpreting perceived human behavior based on intentional mental states such as needs, desires, feelings, beliefs, goals, purposes, and reasons. The term imaginative mental activity indicates that this process is performed by a person using imagination in his/her mind. Mentalizing is a process that enables individuals to correctly understand their own and other people's behavior in interpersonal relationships, as well as to regulate their own emotions and impulses well [60–62].

Capacity for mentalizing the individual develops in childhood and is highly associated with a secure affective attachment to primary caregivers. Mentalizing implies at least the following four dimensions: the first refers to the question of whose behavior is being mentalized - one's own or someone else's; the second refers to the question of the extent to which the individual controls mentalization - at one end it is automatic and implicit, and at the other end of that dimension it is conscious, voluntary or explicit mentalization; the third dimension refers to the use of cognitive and emotional processes, on the one hand there is the possibility to recognize mental phenomena, name and describe their causes and consequences in words, on the other is the possibility to experience these phenomena as feelings without the use of words; the fourth dimension refers to the contents that are mentalized, at one end of this dimension are the contents observed during direct communication with another person, either verbal or nonverbal channel, at the other end are assumptions that depend on the previous experience of the person being mentalizing, which among other things, is influenced by the socio-cultural environment in which that person lives [60–62]. In direct contact with another person, the basic mental actions that an individual performs when mentalizing are to make assumptions about the mental states that determine behavior and check them. Then the individual is aware that intentional mental states cannot be seen with the naked eye. During mentalization, an individual has a not knowing stance about intentional mental states and a sincere curiosity that helps him/her discover them in cooperation with another person [60–62].

Weak capacity for mentalizing has been found in patients with borderline personality disorder, but other mental disorders also include difficulties in mentalization [62, 63]. Also, in the non-clinical population, forms of impaired capacity for mentalizing were examined. Two such forms were investigated in these studies: hypomentalizing and hypermentalizing. These are two qualitatively different phenomena, not extremes of the same [42].

Hypomentalizing refers to the lack or absence of consideration of the phenomena of mental life that determine behavior, and by making assumptions and checking them in interpersonal interaction. Hypomentalizing can be a consequence of a lack of faith in one's own ability to know the mental world, or as a consequence of mistaken beliefs that behavior is determined by external forces, not mental states. Among other things, it manifests as uncertainty in the ability to accurately assess the mental states underlying behavior [61, 64].

Hypermentalizing refers to making too many assumptions about intentional mental states, some of which are uncritically accepted as true, even though they are not true. The hypermentalizing of an individual occurs as a consequence of his/her erroneous beliefs that other persons have identical intentional mental states as himself. It manifests itself as excessive certainty in the accuracy of one's own beliefs about the nature of mental states that underlie one's behavior [61, 64].

There are findings that indicate that a good capacity for mentalizing allows a correct understanding of one's own and others' behavior in stressful situations, which helps to overcome stress [62, 65]. Authors [65] examined the relationship between global distress, capacity for mentalizing and well-being in a sample of German teachers, and found that mentalizing is positively associated with well-being and that mentalizing mitigates the negative impact of stress and psychological symptoms on well-being. In Spain, a study was conducted that examined the association between capacity for mentalizing and burnout syndrome in a sample of entrepreneurs. Research conducted in Spain has shown that the capacity for mentalizing reduces the degree of burnout syndrome in entrepreneurs by reducing emotional exhaustion and cynicism (depersonalization), and that hypomentalizing was a statistically significant positive predictor of emotional exhaustion and cynicism in entrepreneurs [64].

Good capacity for mentalizing is key to resilience - the ability of an individual to return to a state of normal mental functioning after stressful or threatening events, without lasting negative consequences [43]. The first study in the world that linked capacity for mentalizing and resilience to burnout syndrome in a sample of healthcare workers during the COVID-19 pandemic, revealed that there were negative correlations between resilience and burnout dimensions - emotional exhaustion and depersonalization, and positive correlations between resilience and personal achievement. Also, hypomentalizing has been shown to be a significant positive predictor of emotional exhaustion and depersonalization as a dimensions of burnout syndrome [42]. Good capacity for mentalizing means that empathy, active listening and authentic curiosity about mental states, both one's own and the interlocutor's, are expressed during direct communication. Hypomentalizers, instead of revealing objective facts about the reasons for their behavior through open communication with others, usually judge intentional mental states by "guessing", referring to general laws and their previous experience, which leads to wrong conclusions. Lack of mentalizing reduces the ability of people to understand their own and others' behavior, which leads to interpersonal misunderstandings, conflicts, dissatisfaction and professional frustrations. This is consistent with previous findings proving that good mentalizing ability is a protective factor of mental health [60, 63, 64].

Schwarzer et al. [65] found that the presence of stress negatively affected subjective assessments of well-being, while the capacity for mentalizing had an indirect and positive effect on an individual's assessments of health. Evidence suggests that impaired capacity for mentalizing, typical of various mental illnesses, can be improved by psychotherapeutic intervention, leading to a reduction in psychological symptoms [66]. Relying on clinical relevance, there has been a shift towards focusing on capacity for mentalizing as a mediating capacity to promote health in non-clinical populations [60, 62, 63, 65]. Most important in this context is the idea that preventive or early interventions that encourage good capacity for mentalizing can protect the individual from the influence of distress factors [67], thus enabling more resilient adaptation to life stressors and protecting the mental health of the individual.

Concerns about the potential increase in mental disorders have led countries around the world to include psychosocial support in their COVID-19 response plans, among other measures to combat COVID-19, but major shortcomings and concerns remain [68].

## 4. Conclusions

The outbreak of COVID-19 has caused enormous psychological impact worldwide and poses an unprecedented threat to mental health. The extant scientific literature, which reports on mental health status and the prevalence of psychological disorders during the COVID-19 pandemic, warns that the level of depression, anxiety and stress among citizens around the world has reached alarming proportions.

Given that the COVID-19 pandemic marks a global public health crisis unseen in the last century, there is an urgent need to implement measures and strategies to minimize the impact of the COVID-19 pandemic on mental health. As resilience and capacity for mentalizing have been shown to play a very important preventive role when it comes to mental health, it is essential to develop and implement strategies to encourage resilience and strengthen capacity for mentalizing to counteract psychological stress during public health emergencies, including response to COVID-19.

In addition to combating the spread of the Sars-CoV-2 virus, mitigating the devastating effects of COVID-19 on the mental health of both general population and vulnerable groups should be an international public health priority.

This book chapter sought, in addition to reviewing the prevalence of mental disorders during the COVID-19 pandemic and the role of preventive mental health factors such as resilience and good capacity for mentalizing, to emphasize a wake-up call to all countries to pay more attention to mental health and work better to support the mental health of their populations.

## Acknowledgments/notes/thanks

The authors want to thank and dedicate this book chapter to their parents who have always taught them to hope in life and never give up.

## Conflict of interest

The authors declare no conflict of interest.

## Author details

Teodora Safiye[1*], Medo Gutić[1,2], Ardea Milidrag[1], Milena Zlatanović[1] and Branimir Radmanović[1,3]

1 Faculty of Medical Sciences, University of Kragujevac, Kragujevac, Serbia

2 Public Health Institution Health Center “Dr Branko Zogović”, Plav, Montenegro

3 University Clinical Center Kragujevac, Psychiatry Clinic, Kragujevac, Serbia

*Address all correspondence to: teodoras0306@gmail.com

## References

[1] Wu YC, Chen CS, Chan YJ. The outbreak of COVID-19: An overview. Journal of the Chinese Medical Association. 2020;**83**:217-220. DOI:10.1097/JCMA.0000000000000270

[2] Velavan TP, Meyer CG. The COVID-19 epidemic. Tropical Medicine & International Health. 2020;**25**:278-280. DOI: 10.1111/tmi.13383

[3] Vujčić I, Safiye T, Milikić B, Popović E, Dubljanin D, Dubljanin E, et al. Coronavirus disease 2019 (COVID-19) epidemic and mental health status in the general adult population of Serbia: A cross-sectional study. International Journal of Environmental Research and Public Health. 2021;**18**:1957. DOI: 10.3390/ijerph18041957

[4] Galderisi S, Heinz A, Kastrup M, Beezhold J, Sartorius N. Toward a new definition of mental health. World Psychiatry. 2015;**14**:231-233. DOI: 10.1002/wps.20231

[5] Brooks SK, Webster RK, Smith LE, Woodland L, Wessely S, Greenberg N, et al. The psychological impact of quarantine and how to reduce it: Rapid review of the evidence. Lancet. 2020;**395**:912-920. DOI: 10.1016/S0140-6736(20)30460-8

[6] Godoy LD, Rossignoli MT, Delfino-Pereira P, Garcia-Cairasco N, de Lima Umeoka EH. A comprehensive overview on stress neurobiology: Basic concepts and clinical implications. Frontiers in Behavioral Neuroscience. 2018;**12**:127. DOI: 10.3389/fnbeh.2018.00127

[7] Lovibond SH, Lovibond PF. Manual for the Depression Anxiety Stress Scales. 2nd. ed. Sydney: Psychology Foundation; 1995

[8] Xiong J, Lipsitz O, Nasri F, Lui LMW, Gill H, Phan L, et al. Impact of COVID-19 pandemic on mental health in the general population: A systematic review. Journal of Affective Disorders. 2020;**277**:55-64. DOI: 10.1016/j.jad.2020.08.001

[9] Thombs BD, Bonardi O, Rice DB, Boruff JT, Azar M, He C, et al. Curating evidence on mental health during COVID-19: A living systematic review. Journal of Psychosomatic Research. 2020;**133**:110113. DOI: 10.1016/j.jpsychores.2020.110113

[10] Salari N, Hosseinian-Far A, Jalali R, Vaisi-Raygani A, Rasoulpoor S, Mohammadi M, et al. Prevalence of stress, anxiety, depression among the general population during the COVID-19 pandemic: A systematic review and meta-analysis. Globalization and Health. 2020;**16**(1):57. DOI: 10.1186/s12992-020-00589-w

[11] Safiye T, Vukčević B. Dimensions of general psychological distress and age as the predictors of procrastination in university students. Psihološka istraživanja. 2020;**24**:187-200. DOI: 10.5937/PSISTRA23-27810

[12] Odriozola-González P, Planchuelo-Gómez Á, Irurtia MJ, de Luis-García R. Psychological effects of the COVID-19 outbreak and lockdown among students and workers of a Spanish university. Psychiatry Research. 2020;**290**:113108. DOI: 10.1016/j.psychres.2020.113108

[13] Patsali ME, Mousa DV, Papadopoulou EVK, Papadopoulou KKK, Kaparounaki CK, Diakogiannis I, et al. University students' changes in mental health status and determinants of behavior during the COVID-19 lockdown

in Greece. Psychiatry Research. 2020;**292**:113298. DOI: 10.1016/j.psychres.2020.113298

[14] Bourion-Bédès S, Tarquinio C, Batt M, Tarquinio P, Lebreuilly R, Sorsana C, et al. Psychological impact of the COVID-19 outbreak on students in a French region severely affected by the disease: Results of the PIMS-CoV 19 study. Psychiatry Research. 2021;**295**:113559. DOI: 10.1016/j.psychres.2020.113559

[15] Oliveira Carvalho P, Hülsdünker T, Carson F. The impact of the COVID-19 lockdown on European Students' negative emotional symptoms: A systematic review and meta-analysis. Behavior Science (Basel). 2021;**12**:3. DOI: 10.3390/bs12010003

[16] Ajduković D, Rezo Bagarić I, Bakić H, Stevanović A, Frančišković T, Ajduković M. Mental health status and risk factors during Covid-19 pandemic in the Croatia's adult population. European Journal of Psychotraumatology. 2021;**12**:1984050. DOI: 10.1080/20008198.2021.1984050

[17] Kang L, Li Y, Hu S, Chen M, Yang C, Yang BX, et al. The mental health of medical workers in Wuhan, China dealing with the 2019 novel coronavirus. Lancet Psychiatry. 2020;**7**:e14. DOI: 10.1016/S2215-0366(20)30047-X

[18] Xiao X, Zhu X, Fu S, Hu Y, Li X, Xiao J. Psychological impact of healthcare workers in China during COVID-19 pneumonia epidemic: A multi-center cross-sectional survey investigation. Journal of Affective Disorders. 2020;**274**:405-410. DOI: 10.1016/j.jad.2020.05.081

[19] Lai J, Ma S, Wang Y, Cai Z, Hu J, Wei N, et al. Factors associated with mental health outcomes among health care workers exposed to coronavirus disease 2019. JAMA Network Open. 2020;**3**:e203976. DOI: 10.1001/jamanetworkopen.2020.3976

[20] Zerbini G, Ebigbo A, Reicherts P, Kunz M, Messman H. Psychosocial burden of healthcare professionals in times of COVID-19 - a survey conducted at the university hospital Augsburg. Ger. Medical Science. 2020;**18**:Doc05. DOI: 10.3205/000281

[21] Cai Q, Feng H, Huang J, Wang M, Wang Q, Lu X, et al. The mental health of frontline and non-frontline medical workers during the coronavirus disease 2019 (COVID-19) outbreak in China: A case-control study. Journal of Affective Disorders. 2020;**275**:210-215. DOI: 10.1016/j.jad.2020.06.031

[22] Fridner A, Belkic K, Marini M, Sendén MG, Schenck-Gustafsson K. Why don't academic physicians seek needed professional help for psychological distress? Swiss Medical Weekly. 2012;**142**:w13626. DOI: 10.4414/smw.2012.13626

[23] Lv Y, Zhang Z, Zeng W, Li J, Wang X, Luo GQ. Anxiety and depression survey of Chinese medical staff before and during COVID-19 defense. SSRN Electronic Journal. 2020. DOI: 10.2139/ssrn.3551350

[24] Muller AE, Hafstad EV, Himmels JPW, Smedslund G, Flottorp S, Stensland SØ, et al. The mental health impact of the covid-19 pandemic on healthcare workers, and interventions to help them: A rapid systematic review. Psychiatry Research. 2020;**293**:113441. DOI: 10.1016/j.psychres.2020.113441

[25] Ahmed MZ, Ahmed O, Aibao Z, Hanbin S, Siyu L, Ahmad A. Epidemic of COVID-19 in China and associated psychological problems. Asian Journal

of Psychiatry. 2020;**51**:102092. DOI: 10.1016/j.ajp.2020.102092

[26] Gao J, Zheng P, Jia Y, Chen H, Mao Y, Chen S, et al. Mental health problems and social media exposure during COVID-19 outbreak. PLoS One. 2020;**15**:e0231924. DOI: 10.1371/journal.pone.0231924

[27] Lei L, Huang X, Zhang S, Yang J, Yang L, Xu M. Comparison of prevalence and associated factors of anxiety and depression among people affected by versus people unaffected by quarantine during the COVID-19 epidemic in southwestern China. Medical Science Monitor. 2020;**26**:e924609. DOI: 10.12659/MSM.924609

[28] Olagoke AA, Olagoke OO, Hughes AM. Exposure to coronavirus news on mainstream media: The role of risk perceptions and depression. British Journal of Health Psychology. 2020;**25**:865-874. DOI: 10.1111/bjhp.12427

[29] Wang C, Pan R, Wan X, Tan Y, Xu L, Ho CS, et al. Immediate psychological responses and associated factors during the initial stage of the 2019 coronavirus disease (COVID-19) epidemic among the general population in China. International Journal of Environmental Research and Public Health. 2020;**17**:1729. DOI: 10.3390/ijerph17051729

[30] Mazza C, Ricci E, Biondi S, Colasanti M, Ferracuti S, Napoli C, et al. A Nationwide survey of psychological distress among Italian people during the COVID-19 pandemic: Immediate psychological responses and associated factors. International Journal of Environmental Research and Public Health. 2020;**17**:3165. DOI: 10.3390/ijerph17093165

[31] Ozamiz-Etxebarria N, Dosil-Santamaria M, Picaza-Gorrochategui M, Idoiaga-Mondragon N. Stress, anxiety, and depression levels in the initial stage of the COVID-19 outbreak in a population sample in the northern Spain. Cadernos de Saúde Pública. 2020;**36**:e00054020. DOI: 10.1590/0102-311X00054020

[32] Moghanibashi-Mansourieh A. Assessing the anxiety level of Iranian general population during COVID-19 outbreak. Asian Journal of Psychiatry. 2020;**51**:102076. DOI: 10.1016/j.ajp.2020.102076

[33] Serafini G, Parmigiani B, Amerio A, Aguglia A, Sher L, Amore M. The psychological impact of COVID-19 on the mental health in the general population. QJM. 2020;**113**:531-537. DOI: 10.1093/qjmed/hcaa201

[34] Cao W, Fang Z, Hou G, Han M, Xu X, Dong J, et al. The psychological impact of the COVID-19 epidemic on college students in China. Psychiatry Research. 2020;**287**:112934. DOI: 10.1016/j.psychres.2020.112934

[35] Zhang Y, Ma ZF. Impact of the COVID-19 pandemic on mental health and quality of life among local residents in Liaoning Province, China: A cross-sectional study. International Journal of Environmental Research and Public Health. 2020;**17**:2381. DOI: 10.3390/ijerph17072381

[36] Coiro MJ, Watson KH, Ciriegio A, Jones M, Wolfson AR, Reisman J, et al. Coping with COVID-19 stress: Associations with depression and anxiety in a diverse sample of U.S. adults. Current Psychology. 2021;**1-13**. DOI: 10.1007/s12144-021-02444-6 [Epub ahead of print]

[37] Moccia L, Janiri D, Pepe M, Dattoli L, Molinaro M, De Martin V, et al. Affective temperament, attachment style, and the

psychological impact of the COVID-19 outbreak: An early report on the Italian general population. Brain, Behavior, and Immunity. 2020;**87**:75-79. DOI: 10.1016/j.bbi.2020.04.048

[38] Yıldırım M, Arslan G, Özaslan A. Perceived risk and mental health problems among healthcare professionals during COVID-19 pandemic: Exploring the mediating effects of resilience and coronavirus fear. International Journal of Mental Health and Addiction. 2022;**20**:1035-1045. DOI: 10.1007/s11469-020-00424-8

[39] Yıldırım M, Solmaz F. COVID-19 burnout, COVID-19 stress and resilience: Initial psychometric properties of COVID-19 burnout scale. Death Studies. 2022;**46**:524-532. DOI: 10.1080/07481187.2020.1818885

[40] Yıldırım M, Arslan G. Exploring the associations between resilience, dispositional hope, preventive behaviours, subjective well-being, and psychological health among adults during early stage of COVID-19. Current Psychology. 2020:1-11. DOI: 10.1007/s12144-020-01177-2 [Epub ahead of print]

[41] Heath C, Sommerfield A, von Ungern-Sternberg BS. Resilience strategies to manage psychological distress among healthcare workers during the COVID-19 pandemic: A narrative review. Anaesthesia. 2020;**75**:1364-1371. DOI: 10.1111/anae.15180

[42] Safiye T, Vukčević B, Gutić M, Milidrag A, Dubljanin D, Dubljanin J, et al. Resilience, Mentalizing and burnout syndrome among healthcare workers during the COVID-19 pandemic in Serbia. International Journal of Environmental Research and Public Health. 2022;**19**:6577. DOI: 10.3390/ijerph19116577

[43] Smith BW, Dalen J, Wiggins K, Tooley E, Christopher P, Bernard J. The brief resilience scale: Assessing the ability to bounce back. International Journal of Behavioral Medicine. 2008;**15**(3):194-200. DOI: 10.1080/10705500802222972

[44] Herrman H, Stewart DE, Diaz-Granados N, Berger EL, Jackson B, Yuen T. What is resilience? Canadian Journal of Psychiatry. 2011;**56**:258-265. DOI: 10.1177/070674371105600504

[45] Wald J, Taylor S, Asmundson GJ, Jang KL, Stapleton J. LIterature RevIew of Concepts: PsychologIcal ResIlIency (No. DRDC-CR-2006-073). Vancouver: BrItIsh ColumbIa UnIversIty; 2006

[46] Jensen PM, Trollope-Kumar K, Waters H, Everson J. Building physician resilience. Canadian Family Physician. 2008;**54**(5):722-729

[47] Sull A, Harland N, Moore A. Resilience of health-care workers in the UK; a cross-sectional survey. Journal of Occupational Medicine and Toxicology. 2015;**10**:20. DOI: 10.1186/s12995-015-0061-x

[48] Safiye T, Vukčević B, Čabarkapa M. Resilience as a moderator in the relationship between burnout and subjective well-being among medical workers in Serbia during the COVID-19 pandemic. Vojnosanitetski Pregled. 2021;**78**:1207-1213. DOI: 10.2298/VSP210517070S

[49] Wells M, Avers D, Brooks G. Resilience, physical performance measures, and self-perceived physical and mental health in older Catholic nuns. Journal of Geriatric Physical Therapy (2001). 2012;**35**:126-131. DOI: 10.1519/JPT.0b013e318237103f

[50] Poole JC, Dobson KS, Pusch D. Childhood adversity and adult depression: The protective role of psychological resilience. Child Abuse & Neglect. 2017;**64**:89-100. DOI: 10.1016/j.chiabu.2016.12.012

[51] Shapero BG, Farabaugh A, Terechina O, DeCross S, Cheung JC, Fava M, et al. Understanding the effects of emotional reactivity on depression and suicidal thoughts and behaviors: Moderating effects of childhood adversity and resilience. Journal of Affective Disorders. 2019;**245**:419-427. DOI: 10.1016/j.jad.2018.11.033

[52] Howe A, Smajdor A, Stöckl A. Towards an understanding of resilience and its relevance to medical training. Medical Education. 2012;**46**:349-356. DOI: 10.1111/j.1365-2923.2011.04188.x

[53] Mills J, McKimm J. Resilience: Why it matters and how doctors can improve it. British Journal of Hospital Medicine (London, England). 2016;**77**:630-633. DOI: 10.12968/hmed.2016.77.11.630

[54] Harms PD, Brady L, Wood D, Silard A. (2018). Resilience and Well-Being. Handbook of Well-Being. Salt Lake City, UT: DEF Publishers; 2018

[55] García-Izquierdo M, Meseguer de Pedro M, Ríos-Risquez MI, Sánchez MIS. Resilience as a moderator of psychological health in situations of chronic stress (burnout) in a sample of hospital nurses. Journal of Nursing Scholarship. 2018;**50**:228-236. DOI: 10.1111/jnu.12367

[56] Hu D, Kong Y, Li W, Han Q, Zhang X, Zhu LX, et al. Frontline nurses' burnout, anxiety, depression, and fear statuses and their associated factors during the COVID-19 outbreak in Wuhan, China: A large-scale cross-sectional study. EClinicalMedicine. 2020;**24**:100424. DOI: 10.1016/j.eclinm.2020.100424

[57] Skrove M, Romundstad P, Indredavik MS. Resilience, lifestyle and symptoms of anxiety and depression in adolescence: The young-HUNT study. Social Psychiatry and Psychiatric Epidemiology. 2013;**48**(3):407-416. DOI: 10.1007/s00127-012-0561-2

[58] Anyan F, Hjemdal O. Adolescent stress and symptoms of anxiety and depression: Resilience explains and differentiates the relationships. Journal of Affective Disorders. 2016;**203**:213-220. DOI: 10.1016/j.jad.2016.05.031

[59] Batz C, Tay L. Gender differences in subjective well-being. In: Diener E, Oishi S, Tay L, editors. Handbook of well-being. Salt Lake City, UT: DEF Publishers; 2018. p. 2018

[60] Luyten P, Campbell C, Allison E, Fonagy P. The Mentalizing approach to psychopathology: State of the art and future directions. Annual Review of Clinical Psychology. 2020;**16**:297-325. DOI: 10.1146/annurev-clinpsy-071919-015355

[61] Fonagy P, Luyten P, Moulton-Perkins A, Lee YW, Warren F, Howard S, et al. Development and validation of a self-report measure of Mentalizing: The reflective functioning questionnaire. PLoS One. 2016;**11**:e0158678. DOI: 10.1371/journal.pone.0158678

[62] Fonagy P, Luyten P, Allison E, Campbell C. What we have changed our minds about: Part 1. Borderline personality disorder as a limitation of resilience. Borderline Personality Disorder and Emotion Dysregulation. 2017;**4**:11. DOI: 10.1186/s40479-017-0061-9

[63] Bateman A, Campbell C, Luyten P, Fonagy P. A mentalization-based approach to common factors in the treatment of borderline personality disorder. Current Opinion in Psychology. 2018;**21**:44-49. DOI: 10.1016/j.copsyc.2017.09.005

[64] Manzano-García G, Ayala-Calvo JC, Desrumaux P. Entrepreneurs' capacity for Mentalizing: Its influence on burnout syndrome. International Journal of Environmental Research and Public Health. 2020;**18**:3. DOI: 10.3390/ijerph18010003

[65] Schwarzer NH, Nolte T, Fonagy P, Griem J, Kieschke U, Gingelmaier S. The relationship between global distress, mentalizing and well-being in a German teacher sample. Current Psychology. 2021;**1-10**. DOI: 10.1007/s12144-021-01467-3 [Epub ahead of print]

[66] Gagliardini G, Gullo S, Caverzasi E, Boldrini A, Blasi S, Colli A. Assessing mentalization in psychotherapy: First validation of the Mentalization imbalances scale. Research in Psychotherapy. 2018;**21**:339. DOI: 10.4081/ripppo.2018.339

[67] Brugnera A, Zarbo C, Compare A, Talia A, Tasca GA, De Jong K, et al. Self-reported reflective functioning mediates the association between attachment insecurity and well-being among psychotherapists. Psychotherapy Research. 2021;**31**:247-257. DOI: 10.1080/10503307.2020.1762946

[68] Čabarkapa M, Safiye T, Gutić M. Psychosocial stress and risk assessment during the COVID-19 pandemic: Some preliminary thoughts. International Journal of Population Studies. 2022;**8**:1-5. DOI: 10.18063/ijps.v8i2.1335

Chapter 7

# A New Look at Psychological Health and Life Satisfaction: A Quadripartite Model

*Margarida Gaspar de Matos, Cátia Branquinho, Tania Gaspar, Catarina Noronha, Bárbara Moraes, Fábio Botelho Guedes, Ana Cerqueira, Marina Carvalho, Osvaldo Santos, Nuno Neto Rodrigues and Adilson Marques*

**Abstract**

COVID-19 pandemic had a negative impact on adolescents' psychological health. Two national studies were conducted. The DGEEC study included 9 to 18-year-old pupils. The HBSC study (2 waves) included pupils from the 6th, 8th, 10th, 12th grades. For each study, two groups were established based on life satisfaction scores and on psychological symptoms scores, producing four groups. In both studies, the group with high life satisfaction and reduced psychological symptoms had more boys and younger pupils. The group with low life satisfaction and pronounced psychological symptoms comprised more girls and older pupils. In the DGEEC Study, pupils with low life satisfaction and pronounced psychological symptoms were more likely to exhibit other unwellness signs. In the HBSC study, from 2018 to 2022 (with the COVID-19 in between), psychological symptoms increased significantly and life satisfaction decreased, exacerbating inequities. This model allowed to examine the results of DGEEC and HBSC studies under a new perspective comprising four scenarios, offering an innovative viewpoint on adolescents' psychological health. Results also suggest a potential buffering effect of being physically active, adequate sleep, and adequate screen time. This is a powerful message for health and education professionals and policymakers regarding the relevance of health education and promotion.

**Keywords:** pupils, gender, life satisfaction, psychological symptoms, lifestyles, school, quality of life perception, COVID-19

## 1. Introduction

The vulnerabilities associated with the pandemic of COVID-19 have motivated studies reflecting on adolescents, including their physical and psychological health, either through their research or systematic analysis of documents produced by educational and health institutions and researchers [1–6].

There is an agreement in the research about the psychosocial effects of the COVID-19 pandemic on school-aged children and adolescents [7]. Young people reported feeling more lonely and having more depression and anxiety symptoms [8]. Quantitative studies done all over Europe [9–12] confirm this link and show an increase in symptoms of depression, anxiety, and stress.

Tomé and colleagues [13] argue that given the contingencies grounded in the pandemic by COVID-19 (more specifically, social distancing and general confinement/lockdown of the population), young people's psychosocial contexts are considered to have undergone changes that, in turn, generated risks to their psychological health and life satisfaction [3, 10, 12, 14, 15].

The Dual Factor Model [16–18], was used, with some adaptations for its use in population studies, to understand the psychological health of children and adolescents and the associations with their lives and well-being. This model is here referred as "the quadripartite model", as we retained from this model that life satisfaction and psychological symptoms are not opposed in a continuum of two dimensions, but rather four psychological states: Complete Psychological Health (reduced psychological symptoms and high life satisfaction), Incomplete Psychological Health (reduced psychological symptoms and low life satisfaction), Incomplete Psychological Distress (marked psychological symptoms and increased life satisfaction), and Complete Psychological Distress (marked psychological symptoms and low life satisfaction). Complete Psychological Health implies both conditions: high life satisfaction and reduced psychological symptoms, as suggested in the Dual Factor Model [16–18].

To test this model, data from two national studies, the Directorate-General of Education and Science Statistics of the Ministry of Education and the Ministry of Science (DGEEC), and the Health Behaviour in School-aged Children (HBSC) studies, were used for specific analyses. Gender and grade differences (a proxy for age differences) were confirmed in the four groups (complete and incomplete, health and distress). The DGEEC study also analysed how the situation changes with the perception of quality of life and three health behaviours/lifestyles. Considering HBSC, the differences between the 2018 wave (pre-COVID-19 pandemic) and the 2022 wave (post-COVID-19 pandemic) were analysed.

## 2. STUDY 1: the DGEEC study

### 2.1 Methods

#### *2.1.1 Procedures*

The *Psychological Health and Well-Being | School study* (also called the DGEEC study) was done by the Directorate General of Education and Science Statistics, the Directorate General of Education, the National Programme for the Promotion of School Success, Aventura Social Team/ISAMB, the University of Lisbon, the Order of Portuguese Psychologists, and the Calouste Gulbenkian Foundation, with the approval of the Ministry of Education.

Schools and classes were chosen randomly from a national list, and all the ethical procedures, authorisations, and anonymous and voluntary participation were guaranteed. Questionnaires were administered online. Full details are in the final national report of the DGEEC study [4].

#### *2.1.2 Participants*

This study included 4444 pupils ($M$ = 13.39 ± 2.414; Min = 9 e Max = 18), of whom 52.2% are girls. 27.2% of the participants attended the 2nd cycle of schooling, and 72.8% attended lower and upper secondary education.

### 2.2 Instruments

The measures and variables under study are described in **Table 1**.

### 2.3 Statistical analysis and main results

Two groups were created from the measurement of life satisfaction (low—50.3%; high—49.7%) and two groups were created from the evaluation of psychological symptoms (reduced—53.4%; and pronounced—46.6%). In both variables, the median was used as a cut-off point). The combination of four situations resulted in four groups: (1) *Complete Psychological Health*—high life satisfaction and low psychological symptoms (35.6%); (2) *Incomplete Psychological Health*—low life satisfaction and low psychological symptoms (17.7%); (3) *Incomplete Psychological Distress*—high life satisfaction and pronounced psychological symptoms (14.1%); (4) *Complete Psychological Distress*—low life satisfaction and pronounced psychological symptoms (32.6%).

Age and gender differences and differences related to lifestyles and perceptions of quality of life were analysed through Chi-squares or ANOVAS. A significant level was set at $p < .05$.

#### *2.3.1 Gender and age differences*

It was found that boys are significantly more frequent in the group with high life satisfaction and low psychological symptoms (*Complete Psychological Health*). Girls are significantly more frequent in the group with low life satisfaction and strong psychological symptoms (*Complete Psychological Distress*).

It was also found that younger pupils were significantly more frequent in the group *Complete Psychological Health* and older pupils in the group *Complete Psychological Distress.* A gradient was observed with the increase in school grades.

Overall, the percentage of girls reporting psychological symptoms is significantly higher than that of boys, even when they report high life satisfaction. Conversely, the percentage of boys reporting no psychological symptoms is significantly higher than that of girls, even when they report low life satisfaction.

Younger participants are more satisfied with life, whether or not they have pronounced psychological symptoms, and older participants are less satisfied with life, whether or not they have pronounced psychological symptoms.

#### *2.3.2 Lifestyles/health behaviours and quality-of-life perception differences*

Considering other indicators of psychological well-being (perceived quality of life) and health behaviours (sleep time adequacy, physical activity time, and screen time), the pattern described favours pupils in a state of *Complete Psychological Health* (higher quality of life perception, adequate sleep, physical activity, and screen time) and made more vulnerable pupils in a state of *Complete Psychological Distress,* regarding the same behaviours/situations (**Table 2**). Indeed, the gradient highlights the two "extreme" groups, and the "incomplete" situations tend to place themselves in the middle.

| Variables | Category/Items | Min & Max |
|---|---|---|
| Gender | Boy | |
| | Girl | |
| Age | — | Min = 9 & Max = 18 |
| Grade | From 5th to 12th | Min = 5 & Max = 12 |
| Cycle of studies | 2.° cycle | Min = 1 & Max = 2 |
| | Lower and upper secondary education | |
| Cantril—Life satisfaction (HBSC) [19] | 11-step ladder: "The top of the ladder is "10" and represents the best possible life for you, the bottom of the ladder is "0" and represents the worst possible life for you. Right now, where do you think you are on the ladder?" | 0 = worst possible to 10 = best possible |
| HBSC_WHO-5 \| Total [20] HBSC Psychological symptoms (HBSC) [21, 22] | Sadness | 5 lower to 15 higher 1 to 5—Seldom or Never to every day |
| | Irritability | |
| | Nervousness | |
| | Difficulty falling asleep | |
| | Extreme sadness | |
| Physical Activity (HBSC) [21, 22] | In the past 7 days, how many days did you engage in physical activity for at least 60 minutes? | 0 to 7 days |
| Sleep (HBSC) [21, 22] | In general, how many hours do you sleep each night? | 0 to 10 or more hours |
| Screen time (HBSC) [21, 22] | In general, how many hours do you spend each day in front of a screen (TV, mobile phone, computer, tablet? | 0 to 10 or more hours |

**Table 1.**
*Measures and variables under study.*

| | | N | M | SD | F |
|---|---|---|---|---|---|
| Days with 60 min of adequate physical activity | Incomplete Psychological Health | 741 | 3.34 | 1.90 | 39.89*** |
| | Complete Psychological Distress | 1364 | 2.93 | 1.80 | |
| | Complete Psychological Health | 1478 | 3.69 | 1.89 | |
| | Incomplete Psychological Distress | 593 | 3.34 | 1.83 | |
| Sleep (hours of sleep) | Incomplete Psychological Health | 738 | 7.79 | 1.12 | 210.64*** |
| | Complete Psychological Distress | 1356 | 7.12 | 1.31 | |
| | Complete Psychological Health | 1457 | 8.24 | 1.07 | |
| | Incomplete Psychological Distress | 590 | 7.83 | 1.24 | |
| Screen time (hours of screen time) | Incomplete Psychological Health | 737 | 4.62 | 2.39 | 78.16*** |
| | Complete Psychological Distress | 1364 | 5.41 | 2.55 | |
| | Complete Psychological Health | 1471 | 4.00 | 2.35 | |
| | Incomplete Psychological Distress | 591 | 4.76 | 2.57 | |

| | | N | M | SD | F |
|---|---|---|---|---|---|
| HBSC_WHO-5 \| Total Score (out of 5 to 15) | Incomplete Psychological Health | 778 | 15.28 | 4.28 | 885.87*** |
| | Complete Psychological Distress | 1430 | 10.79 | 4.53 | |
| | Complete Psychological Health | 1561 | 18.81 | 3.99 | |
| | Incomplete Psychological Distress | 617 | 15.42 | 4.23 | |

*Note:* *** $p < 0.001$.

**Table 2.**
*Psychological symptoms and life satisfaction, by days of physical activity, hours of sleep, screen time, quality of life—Analysis of variance between groups.*

## 3. STUDY 2—the HBSC study

### 3.1 Methods

#### *3.1.1 Procedures*

The HBSC study network integrated multiple countries in 2018 and 2022. In 2018, 44 countries participated; in 2022, 51 countries participated [22–24]. Participants constitute a representative sample for the school grades under study. Schools and classes were picked at random from a national list. All ethical procedures and permissions were in place, and participation was both anonymous and voluntary. Questionnaires were administered online. Full details with the final national report of the HBSC study in 2018 [22] and 2022 [23].

#### *3.1.2 Participants*

In 2018, 8215 pupils from the 6th (30.7%), 8th (33.7%), 10th (20.8%), and 12th (14.8%) grades participated, with 52.7% being female and a mean age of 14.36 (SD = 2.28). In 2022, 7649 pupils from the 6th (22.4%), 8th (25.4%), 10th (28.1%), and 12th (24.1%) grades responded, with 51.8% being female and a mean age of 15.05 (SD = 2.36). Therefore, considering the 2018 and 2022 HBSC studies, 15,750 pupils were included, 51.8% from the 2018 HBSC study wave and 48.2% from the HBSC 2022 wave, and 53.2% were female.

### 3.2 Instruments

The measures and variables under study are described in **Table 3**.

### 3.3 Statistical analysis and main results

Two groups were created from the measurement of life satisfaction (low—45.4%; high—54.6%), and two groups were created from the evaluation of psychological symptoms (reduced—47.5%; and pronounced—52.5%). In both variables, the median was used as a cut-off point). Four groups were obtained from the combination of the four situations: (1) *Complete Psychological Health*—high life satisfaction and low psychological symptoms (33.4%); (2) *Incomplete Psychological Health*—low life satisfaction and low psychological symptoms (14.1%); (3) *Incomplete Psychological*

| Variables | Category/Items | Min & Max |
|---|---|---|
| Gender | Boy | |
| | Girl | |
| Age | — | Min = 10 & Max = 18 |
| Grade | 6th, 8th, 10th; 12th | Min = 1 & Max = 4 |
| Cantril—Life satisfaction (HBSC) [19] | 11-step ladder: "The top of the ladder is "10" and represents the best possible life for you, the bottom of the ladder is "0" and represents the worst possible life for you. Right now, where do you think you are on the ladder?" | 0 = worst possible to 10 = best possible |
| HBSC Psychological symptoms (HBSC) [21, 22] | Sadness | 1 to 5—Seldom or Never to every day |
| | Irritability | |
| | Nervousness | |
| | Fear | |

*Adapted from [19, 20].*

**Table 3.**
*Measures and variables under study.*

*Distress*—high life satisfaction and pronounced psychological symptoms (21.2%); (4) *Complete Psychological Distress*—low life satisfaction and pronounced psychological symptoms (31.3%).

It was confirmed, as in the previous DGEEC 2022 study, that in the HBSC study (either in 2018 or in 2022), younger pupils and boys were significantly more frequent in the group of complete psychological health and older pupils and girls were significantly more frequent in the group of complete psychological distress. There was also an age/grade gradient, with the situation deteriorating as schooling progresses.

## 4. Discussion

In this application of the Dual Factor Model [16–18], to a population study, it was found that the model helped to explain the distribution of pupils by each of the situations defined by the four conditions.

As observed in previous research, we discovered that, globally, girls present a more disadvantageous situation in terms of their psychological distress [1, 2, 19, 20, 22, 23, 25, 26]. Additionally, we discovered that, globally, older pupils present a more disadvantageous situation concerning their psychological distress [22]. In a study by Yoon et al. [27], it is reaffirmed that adolescents exhibit clear signs of psychological distress as they age, with this trend becoming more prevalent among girls.

The results indicate that, globally, girls are more likely to report symptoms, even when report high life satisfaction. Boys are more likely to report the absence of symptoms, even when they report low life satisfaction. Also, the youngest are the most likely to express life satisfaction, regardless of the presence or absence of pronounced psychological symptoms. The oldest report the lowest levels of life satisfaction, regardless of the presence or absence of pronounced psychological symptoms. This fact demonstrates the need, already mentioned by the original authors [16–18], to take into account not only the extreme situations of "complete health" and "complete

| | |
|---|---|
| *Complete psychological health*<br>• Younger pupils<br>• Boys<br>• Before COVID-19<br>• More physically active<br>• More sleep<br>• More adequate screen time<br>• Better perception of quality of life | *Incomplete psychological health*<br>• Older pupils<br>• Boys |
| *Incomplete psychological distress*<br>• Younger pupils<br>• Girls | *Complete psychological distress*<br>• Older pupils<br>• Girls<br>• After COVID-19<br>• Less physically active<br>• Less sleep<br>• Less adequate screen time<br>• Worst perception of quality of life |

**Table 4.**
*The quadripartite model—the dual factor model [16, 17] adapted [28]—gender and age/grade differences.*

distress" but also the situations in which only one of the situations occurs (reduced psychological symptoms and high life satisfaction or pronounced psychological symptoms with low life satisfaction) (**Table 4**).

Finally, when considering other indicators of psychological well-being (perceived quality of life) and certain health behaviours (adequacy of sleep time, physical activity time, and screen time), we found that this pattern is repeated, favouring pupils in a state of *Complete Psychological Health* and making pupils in a state of *Complete Psychological Distress* more vulnerable.

As suggested by other authors, this study confirms that for a state of complete psychological well-being, both the dimensions of life satisfaction and absence of psychological distress symptoms are essential [16–18]. These same authors suggest that there is a need to consider situations in which only one of the situations occurs (low psychological symptoms and high life satisfaction or pronounced psychological symptoms with low life satisfaction) is present, as results suggest they may be alert to the differential position of gender across educational levels. The data suggest that, throughout schooling, psychological symptoms are most pronounced in girls even when they refer to high life satisfaction, while in boys, there is a decrease in life satisfaction, even without pronounced psychological symptoms. That is, among girls, it is suggested that girls' negative trend with age is from a status of Incomplete Psychological Distress to a Status of Complete Psychological Distress. In contrast, among boys, it is suggested that boys' negative trend with age is from a status of Complete Psychological Health to a Status of Incomplete Psychological Health.

The significance of being physically active, sleeping an adequate number of hours, and using screens in a balanced and moderated manner are three promising ways to increase the odds for boys and girls to grow older in a state of *Complete Psychological Health*. Consistently, longitudinal studies have demonstrated that screen time and sleep duration are associated with less psychological health [29, 30].

In the HBSC study from 2018 to 2022, not only did psychological symptoms increase significantly and life satisfaction decrease, but the gap between girls and boys and between the oldest and the younger seems to have worsened, increasing the health and well-being gap between gender and age groups/grades [22, 23].

Both DGEEC and HBSC studies have some limitations that should be considered. These are self-report studies with a cross-sectional design, which does not allow making inferences of causality. Despite these limitations, the selection of participants was randomised and stratified by administrative region and level of education, with a high number of participants.

## 5. Conclusions

This quadripartite model allows us to delve deeper into the evolution of life satisfaction and perception of psychological symptoms of distress and look at gender and educational level (age) differences from a different perspective.

This four-scenario perspective provides relevant insight into the worsening of the psychological health of adolescents after the COVID-19 pandemic, accentuates the gender differences already identified, alerts in a more refined way to the gender and grade/age differences, and has already had an impact on the recommendations defined and on the ongoing prevention and promotion measures [4].

Several previous studies [1, 2], specifically the recent HBSC 2022 study [20] and the DGEEC 2022 study [4], emphasise the significance of the prevention of psychological distress and the promotion of psychological health and well-being among adolescents in the school contexts integrates the following.

## Conflict of interest

The authors declare no conflict of interest.

## Author details

Margarida Gaspar de Matos[1,2,3*], Cátia Branquinho[1], Tania Gaspar[1,4], Catarina Noronha[1], Bárbara Moraes[1], Fábio Botelho Guedes[1,5], Ana Cerqueira[1,5], Marina Carvalho[6], Osvaldo Santos[1], Nuno Neto Rodrigues[7] and Adilson Marques[1,5]

1 ISAMB, University of Lisbon, Lisbon, Portugal

2 ISPA University Institute, Lisbon, Portugal

3 Portuguese Catholic University, Lisbon, Portugal

4 HEI-Lab, Lusófona University, Lisbon, Portugal

5 Faculty of Human Kinetics, University of Lisbon, Lisbon, Portugal

6 Manuel Teixeira Gomes Higher Institute, Lisbon, Portugal

7 Direção-Geral de Estatísticas da Educação e Ciência, Lisbon, Portugal

*Address all correspondence to: margaridagasparmatos@medicina.ulisboa.pt

## References

[1] Matos MG. Adolescentes: as suas vidas, o seu futuro. Lisboa: Fundação Francisco Manuel dos Santos; 2020

[2] Matos MG. Adolescentes: tudo o que sempre quis saber sobre o que pensam, o que desejam e o que sentem. Lisboa: Oficina do Livro; 2022

[3] Matos MG, Ramalho S, Santos O, Pereira T. A saúde mental dos alunos e dos profissionais na escola: escolas como ecossistemas de bem-estar, saúde e aprendizagem. In: Miguéns M, editor. Estado da Educação: Conselho Nacional de Educação; 2021. pp. 332-341

[4] Matos MG, Branquinho C, Noronha C, Moraes B, Santos O, Carvalho M, et al. Saúde Psicológica e Bem-estar | Observatório de Saúde Psicológica e Bem-estar: Monitorização e Ação. Lisboa: DGEEC; 2022

[5] Matos MG, Wainwright T. COVID-19 and mental health in school-aged children and young people: Thinking ahead while preparing the return to school and to life "as usual". The Psychologist. 2021;**4**(1):1-12. DOI: 10.33525/PPRJ.V4I1.105

[6] World Health Organization. Strengthening Mental Health Promotion. Geneva, Switzerland: World Health Organization; 2022

[7] Ludwig-Walz H, Dannheim I, Pfadenhauer L, Fegert J, Bujard M. Increase of depression among children and adolescents after the onset of the COVID-19 pandemic in Europe: A systematic review and meta-analysis. Child and Adolescent Psychiatry and Mental Health. 2022;**16**(1):109. DOI: 10.1186/s13034-022-00546-y

[8] Branquinho C, Matos MG. More than one year surfing the waves of COVID-19... and now the vaccination: NA. Psico. 2021;**52**(3):e41303. DOI: 10.15448/1980-8623.2021.3.41303

[9] Daniunaite I, Truskauskaite-Kuneviciene I, Thoresen S, Zelviene P, Kazlauskas E. Adolescents amid the COVID-19 pandemic: A prospective study of psychological functioning. Child and Adolescent Psychiatry and Mental Health. 2021;**15**(1):45. DOI: 10.1186/s13034-021-00397-z

[10] Koper N, Creemers H, van Dam L, Stams G, Branje S. Resilience, well-being and informal and formal support in multi-problem families during the COVID-19 pandemic. Child and Adolescent Psychiatry and Mental Health. 2022;**16**(1):103. DOI: 10.1186/s13034-022-00542-2

[11] Orgilés M, Francisco R, Delvecchio E, Espada J, Mazzeschi C, Pedro M, et al. Psychological symptoms in Italian, Spanish and Portuguese youth during the COVID-19 health crisis: A longitudinal study. Child Psychiatry & Human Development. 2022;**53**(5):853-862. DOI: 10.1007/s10578-021-01211-9

[12] Spencer A, Oblath R, Dayal R, Loubeau J, Lejeune J, Sikov J, et al. Changes in psychosocial functioning among urban, school-age children during the COVID-19 pandemic. Child and Adolescent Psychiatry and Mental Health. 2021;**15**(1):73. DOI: 10.1186/s13034-021-00419-w

[13] Tomé G, Branquinho C, Cerqueira A, Matos MG. COVID-19, social distance and adolescents' risk behaviours, well-being and life satisfaction: A proxy study drawn from HBSC study. Análisis y Modificación de Conducta. 2021;**47**:176. DOI: 10.33776/amc.v47i175.4912

[14] Branquinho C, Santos A, Ramiro L, Matos MG. #COVID#BACKTOSCHOOL: Qualitative study based on the voice of Portuguese adolescents. Journal of Community Psychology. 2021;**49**(7):2209-2220. DOI: 10.1002/jcop.22670

[15] Vries J, Horstmann K, Mussel P. Trajectories in life satisfaction before and during COVID-19 with respect to perceived valence and self-efficacy. Current Psychology. 2022;**12**:1-17. DOI: 10.1007/s12144-022-03829-x

[16] Greenspoon P, Saklofske D. Toward an integration of subjective well-being and psychopathology. Social Indicators Research. 2001;**54**(1):81-108. DOI: 10.1023/A:1007219227883

[17] Keyes C. The mental health continuum: From languishing to flourishing in life. Journal of Health and Social Behavior. 2002;**43**:207-222. DOI: 10.2307/3090197

[18] Westerhof G, Keyes C. Mental illness and mental health: The two continua model across the lifespan. Journal of Adult Development. 2010;**17**(2):110-119. DOI: 10.1007/s10804-009-9082-y

[19] Cantril H. The Pattern of Human Concerns. New Brunswick, NJ, USA: Rutgers University Press; 1965

[20] World Health Organization. Wellbeing Measures in Primary Health Care/the DEPCARE Project: Report on a WHO Meeting. Stockholm, Sweden: World Health Organization; 1998

[21] Inchley J, Currie D, Young T, Samdal O, Torsheim T, Auguston L, Barnekon V. Growing up unequal: gender and socioeconomic differences in young people's health and well-being. Health Behaviour in School-aged Children (HBSC) study: international report from the 2013/2014 survey. World Health Organization (WHO) Regional Office for Europe. 2016

[22] Matos MG, Equipa Aventura Social. A Saúde dos Adolescentes Portugueses após a recessão. Relatório do estudo Health Behaviour in School Aged Children (HBSC) em 2018 (ebook). Lisboa; 2018

[23] Gaspar T, Guedes F, Cerqueira A, Matos MG, Equipa Aventura Social. A saúde dos adolescentes portugueses em contexto de pandemia. Relatório do estudo Health Behaviour in School Aged Children (HBSC) em 2022 (ebook). Lisboa; 2022. Available from: https://aventurasocial.com/dt_portfolios/a-saude-dos-adolescentes-portugueses-em-tempos-de-recessao-2018-2/

[24] Inchley J, Currie D, Budisavljevic S, Torsheim T, Jåstad A, Cosma A, Weber M. Spotlight on adolescent health and well-being. Findings from the 2017/2018 Health Behaviour in School-aged Children (HBSC) survey in Europe and Canada. World Health Organization (WHO) Regional Office for Europe; 2020

[25] Gaspar T, Cerqueira A, Branquinho C, Matos MG. Dimensions of social and personal skills in children and adolescents: Age and gender differences. International Journal of Development Research. 2018;**8**(1):18394-18400

[26] Gaspar T, Tomé G, Gómez-Baya D, Guedes F, Cerqueira A, Borges A, et al. O bem-estar e a saúde mental dos adolescentes portugueses. Revista de Psicologia da Criança e do adolescente. 2019;**10**(1):17-28

[27] Yoon Y, Eisenstadt M, Lereya ST, Deighton J. Gender difference in the change of adolescents' mental health and subjective wellbeing trajectories. European Child & Adolescent Psychiatry. 2022;**2022**:1-10

[28] Matos MG, Branquinho C, Noronha C, Moraes B, Santos O, Carvalho M, Rodrigues N. Modelo quadripartido das relações entre satisfação com a vida e de mal-estar psicológico: potencial impacto nas políticas públicas. In: Matos MG, Branquinho C, Rodrigues N, coordinators. Saúde Psicológica e Bem-estar | Observatório de Saúde Psicológica e Bem-estar: Monitorização e Ação. DGEEC; 2023. p.Error: Reference source not found-251

[29] Li X, Buxton OM, Lee S, Chang AM, Berger LM, Hale L. Sleep mediates the association between adolescent screen time and depressive symptoms. Sleep Medicine. 2019;**57**:51-60

[30] Vandendriessche A, Chekiere A, Van Cauwenberg J, De Clercq B, Dhondt K, DeSmet A, et al. Does sleep mediate the association between school pressure, physical activity, screen time, and psychological symptoms in early adolescents? A 12-Country Study. International Journal of Environmental Research and Public Health. 2019;**16**(6):1072. DOI: 10.1007/s10804-009-9082-y

Chapter 8

# Benefits and Barriers of Physical Activity in Social Inclusion and Quality of Life in People with Serious Mental Disorders

*Cristina Méndez-Aguado, Adolfo J. Cangas, María Jesús Lirola, Juan Leandro Cerezuela and Andrés López-Pardo*

## Abstract

This book chapter presents a review of the main benefits that the practice of physical activity brings to people with severe mental disorder (SMD), as well as highlighting the most significant barriers that hinder their adherence. In this regard, it should be noted that this is a population sector in which sedentary lifestyle habits predominate, showing that physical activity is not only beneficial for physical health but also for mental and social health. However, people with severe mental disorder face barriers in which personal, social, and intervention program factors play a role, what makes regular practice difficult for them and, therefore, to access the numerous benefits it brings.

**Keywords:** Severe mental disorder, physical activity, benefits, barriers, inclusion

## 1. Introduction

Severe mental disorder (SMD) refers to different psychopathological conditions, such as severe depression, bipolar disorder, schizophrenia, or severe personality disorders, which have a duration of at least 2 years and affect several aspects of the person's life (social, clinical, educational, judicial, etc.) [1, 2]. Due to their high impact on quality of life and their current prevalence, they are considered as one of the major health issues [3]. These are people who, for instance, see their life expectancy reduced by 10–20 years [1].

These individuals are at increased risk of medical problems, mainly associated with sedentary lifestyles, poor dietary habits, and the adverse physical and mental effects of toxic intake or medication effects. Possible secondary medical complications include cardiovascular complications, metabolic syndrome, and the development of diabetes [4, 5].

Among the recommendations to palliate these difficulties, the practice of physical activity stands out, as it has benefits not only on physical but also on personal



IntechOpen

well-being and mental health [6, 7]. Through this practice, cardiometabolic complications are affected [8, 9], as well as psychological factors such as mood, self-esteem, and psychological and social well-being, which is also closely related to another common problem in this field, such as stigma toward mental health problems [10].

However, despite the fact that this is a problem with a high incidence among the current population, there are not many studies that focus specifically on the effect of physical activity on people with SMD. This is a topic that has not been formally studied and is mostly based on interventions without follow-up or carried out for short periods of time (1 to 3 months), making it difficult to identify long-term benefits and barriers. Therefore, despite its relevance, there is still a predominant lack of justification for its transfer to clinical routines.

In that sense, this chapter presents a review of the existing literature, with the aim of determining the factors that have a positive effect on the practice of physical activity, as well as the barriers that people with SMD have to face so as to do it. For this purpose, specific attention will be paid to those physical activity programs that have been actively implemented in this population sector, being able to extract the relevant data from them thanks to their empirical analyses, based on the collection of qualitative and quantitative data.

## 2. Benefits

One of the characteristics of the population with some type of SMD is the reduction in the level of quality of life. This has been defined by the World Health Organization [11] as a personal perception, based on the objectives, standards, concerns, and expectations of each individual, of the position they occupy in life according to the cultural environment and the value system established at the time of measurement. In order to quantify this broad concept, six main factors must be addressed: physical health, psychological state, level of dependence, social relations, personal beliefs, and the relationship with the environment.

Of all these factors, three stand out for having been directly analyzed in the available studies on the implementation of physical activity programs for people with SMD. These factors are physical health, mental health, and social relationships, and the benefits obtained in these studies promote the recommendation of physical activity for people with SMD in all clinical intervention guidelines. However, it should be noted that the WHO currently recommends at least 150 minutes of aerobic physical activity per week at a moderate or vigorous intensity in order to obtain significant results, guidelines followed by the studies analyzed for the benefits described in the following section.

### 2.1 Physical health

The contributions of the programs examined in the area of physical health, understood as the link between well-being and proper bodily functioning, have been various.

Applying WHO recommendations, the regular practice of physical activity has been directly and significantly related to improvements in anthropometric measurements, functional fitness, and motor skills of participants. This is due not only to the individual effect on each of these variables but also to the interrelationship between them. Anthropometric measurements include body weight and body circumference and are related to the nutritional and health status of the participants. Their in-depth analysis not only allows predictions to be made about users' performance but also about their health and even survival. At the same time, changes in anthropometric measurements lead to changes in body composition which, together with muscular strength, cardiorespiratory endurance, flexibility, and balance are the main components of functional fitness, as well as motor qualities for which benefits have been proven in different studies [12, 13].

However, physical health is not only related to physical fitness but also to the development of healthy eating and consumption habits. These habits are particularly relevant among people with SMD as, due to medication and the symptoms of the disorder itself, they tend to have a greater appetite and have diets that are low in fruit and vegetables but high in fat and sugar. Physical activity programs have reported improvements in this area by combining physical exercise with educational workshops on healthy behaviors, improving participants' diets and promoting the abandonment of substance, alcohol, and tobacco use, which reduces the possibility of developing diseases related to unhealthy habits [14].

All these improvements, both in terms of physical fitness and eating habits, promote the improvement of the autonomy of this sector of the population. Although this is also influenced by the social aspect, the physical sphere plays a very important role [15]. Improved anthropometric measurements, functional fitness, and motor skills allow for better performance of daily activities, without the need for assistance and/or support. In addition, the inclusion of healthy eating habits and the reduction or cessation of substance, alcohol, and tobacco use also contribute positively, as they do not require supervision in this regard and prevent the occurrence of related health problems.

### 2.2 Mental health

Physical activity programs for people with SMD have also reported various benefits in terms of mental health, understood as a state of being aware of one's individual capacities and being able to face everyday difficulties, work productively, and contribute to the community of which one is a part.

Several authors have focused their studies in this area, determining the improvement of factors such as self-esteem, stress, and anxiety [16, 17]. Similarly, in other work where the effect of a regular football league on mental health was evaluated, they also found improvements in self-stigma [18]. Even in studies where mental health status has been measured in a general way, mental health status has improved equally [19]. Physical activity allows participants to create new goals that they are capable of achieving, giving them the confidence that they can achieve what they set out to do and feel that they contribute to the community in some way. In this way, the perception of self-worth is positively modified while increasing self-esteem and self-image, thus promoting improved mental health.

Likewise, several authors have found significant improvements in symptomatology, both positive and negative, in SMD [20–22] that is addressed through the practice of physical activity thanks to the contributions of this type of activity. On the one hand, the hormonal release that is produced intervenes in the reduction of symptoms related to certain disorders, such as depression or anxiety. On the other hand, the possibility it offers in terms of disconnection also plays a positive role. Users have the opportunity to disconnect the mind by focusing on the task at hand, reducing the attention on negative symptoms that are occurring.

Therefore, physical activity programs develop positive expectations toward symptom improvement so that adherence to such programs is increased [23]. However, the need to control the energy used in physical activity is demonstrated, given that excess energy can also lead to problems in adaptation and behavioral problems [24].

Likewise, in other study proposed, it can be observed how the practice of regular physical activity from an early age acts as a protective factor in various psychological problems, such as depression by acting on all the factors studied earlier [25].

### 2.3 Social relationships

Although there are few practical studies that have directly measured how physical activity affects interactions between two or more people involving a set of implicit norms, they have demonstrated benefits for participants.

In terms of the benefits of physical activity on a social level, some studies highlight improvements in personal and social functioning [12], allowing for the emergence of positive social relationships, reducing self-stigma, all thanks to the contact established during the activity sessions, both between people with SMD and those who do not have SMD [16]. Therefore, the socialization of this group is promoted [15], in which fun acts as a common thread, leading to a reduction in stereotypes and symptomatology and the creation of bonds between those involved [26]. In this way, the practice of physical activity may be a suitable way to improve social support for people with SMD [17].

These improvements appear indirectly, i.e. it does not seem to be necessary for physical activity programs to devote part of the session to this task. In fact, these are benefits detected through studies whose objectives were physical and mental health variables, in which no improvements were obtained, but which were nevertheless positively valued by the participants in view of the social possibilities presented [27].

The internal characteristics of team activities, especially when they are carried out in groups, and the wide range of possibilities they offer, allow participants to value them positively by fostering positive experiences through the exchange of sessions with like-minded people. Team activities offer a wide range of social opportunities by allowing interaction between participants, both during the activity itself, which requires cooperation, and after the activity has ended, and by encouraging the emergence of positive stimulus from other users who are in the same situation.

## 3. Barriers

However, despite all these benefits, the practice of physical activity continues to be a pending subject in this population, possibly due to different barriers, that is to say, elements that hinder participation and continuation in programs of this type. These barriers can be classified into three main groups: personal, social, and/or related to the activity program itself.

### 3.1 Personal barriers

Regarding this type of factors, a study points to the importance of lack of motivation and fatigue [28], to which other researchers add poor physical self-awareness that leads to shortcomings at the motivational level as it predetermines poor performance and performance in physical activity [29]. To these variables, some authors add their own emotional influences [30], closely related to low mood and the presence of high levels of stress [31]. Another research also includes low self-efficacy and stigma [32]. Although it has previously been concluded that these variables are reduced or even eliminated, their existence hinders adherence to physical activity programs and thus the possibility of eliminating them and accessing the benefits they bring.

Along the same lines, it is established as a barrier the personal experience with the disorder, taking into account the symptoms of the disorder and the side effects of medication [33]. To this, together with negative expectations and an incorrect body perception, we must add the achievement of immediate negative results and the misconceptions evoked toward the sport practice itself (type of activity, intensity, etc.) [23].

However, these are barriers that can be overcome by providing the right support to the participants, both during, before, and after the tasks. In this way, the creation of false expectations would be avoided and the demotivation inherent in their nonachievement would be easier to counteract. Such support should come from the relationships established between the providers of the intervention, as well as from the rest of those involved in the program. This would require coordination between all those involved, although this is a barrier that is still present today [34].

### 3.2 Social barriers

The existence of certain social conditioning factors also plays an important role, such as a clear lack of support, both at family and social level and from the health system itself [33]. Thus, according to other studies, the lack of medical staff involved during the development of physical activity is considered a barrier to its practice, since it is interpreted as a lack of support from the environment and increases demotivation [21, 29]. This is a sector of the population that requires more support from their environment to adhere to this type of activities, facing the personal barriers they face.

It is highlighted the shortcomings at the organizational level. On the one hand, they highlight the lack of staff during the development of the physical activity, resulting in difficulties at the level of supervision and, therefore, of individual adaptation of the activity itself, as well as in the absence of guidance and support. On the other hand, they highlight the usual lack of financial resources, not only at an organizational level for these programs, but also at a personal level. These are people with greater economic difficulties that affect the possibilities of accessing sports facilities and acquiring adequate material [35].

### 3.3 Program barriers

With regard to the constraints related to the physical activity program itself, environmental restrictions, lack of staff and support in supervising the implementation of the activities, and the presence of rigid structures that limit spontaneous exercise, that is to say, preestablished exercise site conditions that allow for few changes, are identified [24]. The existence of such structures and the lack of support result in a lack of adaptation of the activities to be performed, which is considered another barrier to be taken into account [21].

At the same time, the lack of appropriate equipment is also seen as a barrier. Currently, the logistical factors of these interventions are characterized by being mostly deficient and not adapted to the needs of the participants or needing to be provided by the participants themselves, a sector of the population with economic deficiencies. This not only leads to lower participation but also contributes to feelings of insecurity during the activities [36].

On the other hand, there is a notable lack of physical activity programs that include and consider the participation of people with severe mental disorder (SMD) [26]. There is insufficient support from previous physical activity programs that could serve as a reference and motivation for both the organizers and the participants themselves. Thus, participation is diminished, as well as the creation of interventions that consider the inclusion of this population.

## 4. Conclusions

The review of the literature carried out throughout this work has allowed us to develop the main objective established, which was to identify the benefits reported by the practice of physical activity for people with SMD and the barriers that act as a hindrance to its implementation.

The results obtained reveal that the practice of physical activity in people suffering from some type of SMD has many benefits. It allows for an improvement in physical fitness, whether in terms of anthropometric measurements or physical condition, and facilitates the acquisition of healthy habits, thereby reducing the likelihood of developing diseases related to unhealthy habits, such as smoking or a sedentary lifestyle [37]. This is of great relevance as it aims to reduce certain health risk factors identified by the World Health Organization as the main causes of death from cardiovascular problems, placing it at around 61% of total deaths [38].

In terms of mental health, this also benefits as the practice of physical activity intervenes on psychological problems such as self-esteem, stress, or anxiety. The development of these factors is of great importance as it contributes positively to the improvement of autonomy [39]. This improvement also contributes to the reduction of the symptoms of the disorder, as stated by Stubbs. This reduction in symptomatology could lead to a reduction in the consumption of drugs, together with the benefits of sport on certain health problems derived from the side effects of the medication prescribed for the disorder in question [40].

Other reported benefits are related to social factors. The studies analyzed have found that the practice of physical activity promotes socialization and the development of social relationships, which acts against the usual isolation in this population [41].

Nevertheless, it should be noted that, despite the potential negative impact and recommendations due to the benefits found, people with SMD often do not engage in any type of physical activity [42]. Low adherence is prevalent and needs to be corrected to achieve significant results as regular practice is important [43]. This lack of adherence is due, in part, to the presence of various barriers that need to be addressed. According to those found throughout the literature review, these include personal, social, and program-specific factors.

Regarding the former, the main stumbling block to consider is demotivation toward this practice. This may be related to various factors, such as a low self-concept, fatigue, erroneous beliefs about individual abilities and skills, and even negative emotional influence caused by stress or low mood. These problems are derived from the physical inactivity itself or appear as a consequence of the disorder or as side effects of the pharmacological treatment administered [39, 44, 45].

There are also barriers around the physical activity program itself. These lie in logistical factors such as lack of equipment, lack of support from physical activity specialists, and nonstandardized locations, i.e. limitations intrinsic to the facilities in which the activity takes place. These barriers contribute to demotivation due to the difficulties of access that they entail [32].

In terms of social factors, two main ones stand out. On the one hand, the lack of support from the environment and, on the other hand, the problems derived from the healthcare system. In this regard, the lack of training and awareness in this regard both on the part of the immediate environment and healthcare staff stands out [32]. Similarly, the current healthcare system gives greater importance to pharmacological treatment [46], leaving other types of interventions such as physical activity in the background.

## Acknowledgements

This work has been financed with the support of a project of the Andalusian Knowledge Agency (P20_00232).

## Author details

Cristina Méndez-Aguado[1], Adolfo J. Cangas[2*], María Jesús Lirola[2], Juan Leandro Cerezuela[1] and Andrés López-Pardo[3]

1 Department of Education, University of Almería, Almería, Spain

2 Department of Psychology, University of Almería, Almería, Spain

3 Andalusian Public Foundation for the Social Integration of People with Schizophrenia (FAISEM), Sevilla, Spain

*Address all correspondence to: ajcangas@ual.es

## References


[1] Liu NH, Daumit GL, Dua T, Aquila R, Charlson F, Cuijpers P, et al. Excess mortality in persons with severe mental disorders: A multilevel intervention framework and priorities for clinical practice, policy and research agendas. World Psychiatry. 2017;**16**:30-40. DOI: 10.1002/wps.20384

[2] National Institute of Mental Health. Towards a model for a comprehensive community based mental health system. Washington DC: NIMH; 1987

[3] Marco A. Programa de promoción de hábitos de vida saludable para personas con trastorno mental grave en una unidad de salud mental comunitaria. Revista de Enfermería en Salud Mental. 2020;**14**:20-24. DOI: 10.5538/2385-703X.2020.14.20

[4] Das-Munshi J, Chang C-K, Dutta R, Morgan C, Nazroo J, Stewart R, et al. Ethnicity and excess mortality in severe mental illness: A cohort study. Lancet Psychiatry. 2017;**4**:389-399. DOI: 10.1016/S2215-0366(17)30097-4

[5] Martín, G. El deporte como tratamiento no farmacológico de la enfermedad mental. In: Proyecto MENS editors. 12 artículos que conectan salud mental con deporte y actividad física. Brussels: ENALMH; 2018. p. 107-118

[6] Holt NL. Positive Youth Development Through Sport. Abingdon: Routledge; 2016

[7] Schuch FB, Vancampfort D, Firth J, Rosenbaum S, Ward PB, Silva ES, et al. Physical activity and incident depression: A meta-analysis of prospective cohort studies. The American Journal of Psychiatry. 2018;**175**:631-648. DOI: 10.1176/appi.ajp.2018.17111194

[8] Correll CU, Solmi M, Veronese N, Bortolato B, Rosson S, Santonastaso P, et al. Prevalence, incidence and mortality from cardiovascular disease in patients with pooled and specific severe mental illness: A large-scale meta-analysis of 3,211,768 patients and 113,383,368 controls. World Psychiatry. 2017;**16**:163-180. DOI: 10.1002/wps.20420

[9] Vancampfort D, Stubbs B, Mitchell AJ, De Hert M, Wampers M, Ward PB, et al. Risk of metabolic syndrome and its components in people with schizophrenia and related psychotic disorders, bipolar disorder and major depressive disorder: A systematic review and meta-analysis. World Psychiatry. 2015;**14**:339-347. DOI: 10.1002/wps.20252

[10] Vaca S, Martínez JM. Análisis del estigma hacia personas con trastorno mental grave en la población de Cáceres. Revista de Educación Social. 2019;**29**:142-153

[11] WHOQOL Group. The World Health Organization Quality of life assessment (WHOQOL). Position Paper from the World Health Organization. Social Science & Medicine. 1995;**41**(10): 1.403-1.409

[12] Mullor D, Gallego J, Cangas AJ, Aguilar-Parra JM, Valenzuela L, Mateu JM, et al. Efectividad de un programa de actividad física en personas con trastorno mental grave/effectiveness of a program of physical activity in people with serious mental disorder. Revista Internacional de Medicina y Ciencias de la Actividad Física y el Deporte. 2017;**17**:507-521. DOI: 10.15366/rimcafd2017.67.008

[13] Pérez-Cruzado D, Cuesta-Vargas AI, Vera-García E, Mayoral-Cleries F.

Physical fitness and levels of physical activity in people with severe mental illness: A cross-sectional study. BMC Sports Science, Medicine and Rehabilitation. 2017;**9**:1-6. DOI: 10.1186/s13102-017-0082-0

[14] Smith J, Griffiths LA, Band M, Hird-Smith R, Williams B, Bold J, et al. Early intervention in psychosis: Effectiveness and implementation of a combined exercise and health behavior intervention within routine care. Frontiers in Endocrinology. 2020;**11**:1-19. DOI: 10.3389/fendo.2020.577691

[15] Guérin E, Dupuis J-P, Jacob J-D, Prud'homme D. Incorporating a physical activity program into an assertive community treatment team: Impact and strategies. Community Mental Health Journal. 2019;**55**:1293-1297. DOI: 10.1007/s10597-019-00440-6

[16] Galán-Casado D, Castillo J, García B. Deporte e inclusión social en personas con trastorno mental grave (TMG). Psychology, Society and Education. 2020;**12**:71-83. DOI: 10.25115/psye.v10i1.2343

[17] Young D, Yat-Nam P, Cheng D, Hong LC. Effects of physical activity intervention for Chinese people with severe mental illness. Research on Social Work Practice. 2019;**29**:796-807. DOI: 10.1177/1049731518804900

[18] Moraleda A, Galán-Casado D, Cangas AJ. Reducing self-stigma in people with severe mental illness participating in a regular football league: An exploratory study. International Journal of Environmental Research and Public Health. 2019;**16**:3599. DOI: 10.3390/ijerph16193599

[19] Battaglia G, Alesi M, Inguglia M, Roccella M, Caramazza G, Bellafiore M, et al. Soccer practice as an add-on treatment in the management of individuals with diagnosis of schizophrenia. Neuropsychiatric Disease and Treatment. 2013;**9**:595-603. DOI: 10.2147/NDT.S44066

[20] Firth J, Carney R, Pownall M, French P, Elliott R, Cotter J, et al. Challenges in implementing an exercise intervention within residential psychiatric care: A mixed methods study. Mental Health and Physical Activity. 2017;**12**:141-146. DOI: 10.1016/j.mhpa.2017.04.004

[21] Kinnafick F-E, Papathomas A, Regoczi D. Promoting exercise behavior in a secure mental health setting: Healthcare assistant perspectives. International Journal of mental Health Nursing. 2018;**27**:1776-1783. DOI: 10.1111/inm.12484

[22] Mullor D, Cangas AJ, Gallego J, Trigueros R, López A. Impacto psicológico y social de un programa de deporte inclusivo entre estudiantes y personas con trastorno mental grave. Revista de Psicología del Deporte. 2020;**29**:5-15

[23] Rastad C, Martin C, Asenlöf P. Barriers, benefits and strategies for physical activity in patients with schizophrenia. Psyhical Therapy. 2014;**94**:1467-1479. DOI: 10.2522/ptj.20120443

[24] Rogers E, Papathomas A, Kinnafick F-E. Inpatient perspectives on physical activity in a secure mental health setting. Psychology of Sport and Exercise. 2021;**52**:101827. DOI: 10.1016/j.psychsport.2020.101827

[25] Nietola M, Huovinen H, Heiskala A, Nordström T, Miettunen J, Korkeila J, et al. Early childhood and adolescent risk factors for psychotic depression in a general population birth cohort

sample. Social Psychiatry and Psychiatric Epidemiology. 2020;**55**:1179-1186. DOI: 10.1007/s00127-020-01835-7

[26] Brooke LE, Gucciardi DF, Ntoumanis N, Lin A. Qualitative investigation of perceived barriers to and enablers of sport participation for young people first episode psychosis. Early Intervention in Psychiatry. 2019;**14**:293-306. DOI: 10.1111/eip.12854

[27] Walburg FS, de Joode JW, Brandt HE, van Tulder MW, Adriaanse MC, van Meijel B. Implementation of a lifestyle intervention for people with severe mental illness (SMILE): A process evaluation. BMC Health Services Research. 2022;**22**:1-12. DOI: 10.1186/s12913-021-07391-3

[28] Romain AJ, Longpré-Poirier C, Tannous M, Abdel-Baki A. Physical activity for patients with severe mental illness: Preferences, barriers and perceptions of counselling. Science and Sports. 2020;**35**:289-299. DOI: 10.1016/j.scispo.2020.03.005

[29] Yap J, McCartan C, Davidson G, White C, Bradley L, Webb P, et al. An exercise intervention for people with serious mental illness: Findings from a qualitative data analysis using participatory theme elicitation. Health Expectations. 2020;**23**:1579-1593. DOI: 10.1111/hex.13141

[30] Matthews E, Cowman M, Brannigan M, Sloan D, Ward PB, Denieffe S. Examining the barriers to physical activity between active and inactive people with severe mental illness in Ireland. Mental Health and Physical Activity. 2018;**15**:139-144. DOI: 10.1016/j.mhpa.2018.10.003

[31] Firth J, Rosenbaum S, Stubbs B, Gorcynski P, Yung AR, Vancampfort D. Motivating factors and barriers towards exercise in severe mental illness: A systematic review ad meta-analysis. Psychological Medicine. 2016;**46**:2869-2881. DOI: 10.1017/S0033291716001732

[32] Chen M-D, I J-H, Pellegrini CA, Tang T-C, Kuo C-C. A qualitative exploration of facilitators and barriers to physical activity participation in people with severe mental illness in Taiwan. Mental Health and Physical Activity. 2017;**13**:100-107. DOI: 10.1016/j.mhpa.2017.09.004

[33] Rezaie L, Shafaroodi N, Philips D. The barriers to participation in leisure time physical activities among Iranian women with severe mental illness: A qualitative study. Mental Health and Physical Activity. 2017;**13**:171-177. DOI: 10.1016/j.mhpa.2017.09.008

[34] Melamed OC, Fernando I, Soklaridis S, Hahn MK, LeMessurier KW, Taylor VH. Understanding engagement with a physical health service: A qualitative study of patients with severe mental illness. The Canadian Journal of Psychiatry. 2019;**64**:872-880. DOI: 10.1177/0706743719862980

[35] Deenik J, Tenback DE, Tak ECPM, Henkemans OAB, Rosenbaum S, Hendriksen IJM, et al. Implementation barriers and facilitators of an integrated multidisciplinary lifestyle enhancing treatment for inpatients with severe mental illness: The MULTI study IV. Health Service Research. 2019;**19**:1-13. DOI: 10.1186/s12913-019-4608-x

[36] Martland R, Gaughran F, Stubbs B, Onwumere J. Perspectives on implementing HIIT interventions for service users in inpatient mental health settings: A qualitative study investigating patient, carer and staff attitudes. Journal of Affective Disorders. 2021;**283**:198-206. DOI: 10.1192/bjo.2021.716

[37] Mullor D, Cangas AJ, Gallego J, Aguilar R, A., López, A. A longitudinal study about the impact of an inclusive sports program in people with diagnosis of schizophrenia. Psychosis - Psychological Social and Integrative Approaches. 2019;**11**:75-84. DOI: 10.1080/17522439.2018.1559873

[38] World Health Organization. Global Health Risks: Mortality and Burden of Disease Attributable to Selected Major Risks. Geneva: World Health Organization; 2009

[39] Pereira CS, Padoan CS, García LF, Patusco L, Magalhães PVS. Barreras y facilitadores percibidos por personas con trastorno bipolar para la práctica del ejercicio: Un estudio cualitativo. Tendencias Psiquiatría Psicoterapeuta. 2019;**41**:1-8

[40] Stubbs B, Vancampfort D, Hallgren M, Firth J, Veronese N, Solmi M, et al. EPA guidance on physical activity as a treatment for severe mental illness: A meta-review of the evidence and Position Statement from the European Psychiatric Association (EPA), supported by the International Organization of Physical Therapists in Mental Health (IOPTMH). European Psychiatry. 2018;**54**:124-144. DOI: 10.1016/j.eurpsy.2018.07.004

[41] Hargreaves J, Lucock M, Rodriguez A. From inactivity to becoming physically active: The experiences of behaviour change in people with serious mental illness. Mental Health and Physical Activity. 2017;**13**:83-93. DOI: 10.1016/j.mhpa.2017.09.006

[42] Ashdown-Franks G, Williams J, Vancampfort D, Firth J, Schuch F, Hubbard K, et al. Is it possible for people with severe mental illness to sit less and move more? A systematic review of interventions to increase physical activity or reduce sedentary behavior. Schizophrenia Research. 2018;**202**:3-16. DOI: 10.1016/j.schres.2018.06.058

[43] Barton J, Rogerson M. The importance of greenspace for mental health. British Journal of Psychiatry International. 2017;**14**:79-81. DOI: 10.1192/s2056474000002051

[44] Ballesteros N, Moruno P. Análisis descriptivo de la actividad física en personas con enfermedad mental que asisten a Centros de Rehabilitación Psicosocial y Laboral en Castilla La-Mancha. Estudio Piloto. Revista Electrónicas de Terapia Ocupacional Galicia. 2012;**9**:1-27

[45] Shor R, Shalev A. Barriers to involvement in physical activities of persons with mental illness. Health Promotion International. 2016;**31**:116-123. DOI: 10.1093/heapro/dau078

[46] Mugisha J, De Hertc M, Knizekd BL, Kwiringiraa J, Kinyandae E, Byansil W, et al. Health care professionals' perspectives on physical activity within the Ugandan mental health care system. Mental Health and Physical Activity. 2019;**16**:1-7. DOI: 10.1016/j.mhpa.2019.02.001